Reproductive Biology and Technology in Animals

Edited by Juan Carlos Gardón Poggi and Katy Satué Ambrojo

Published in London, United Kingdom

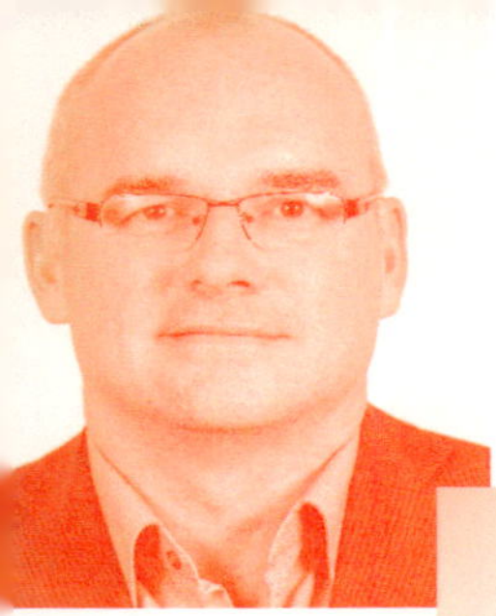
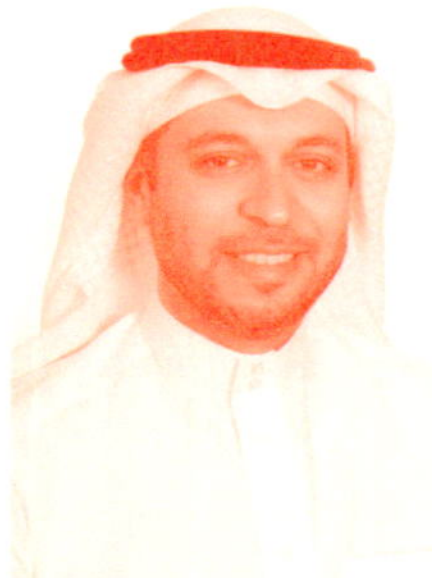
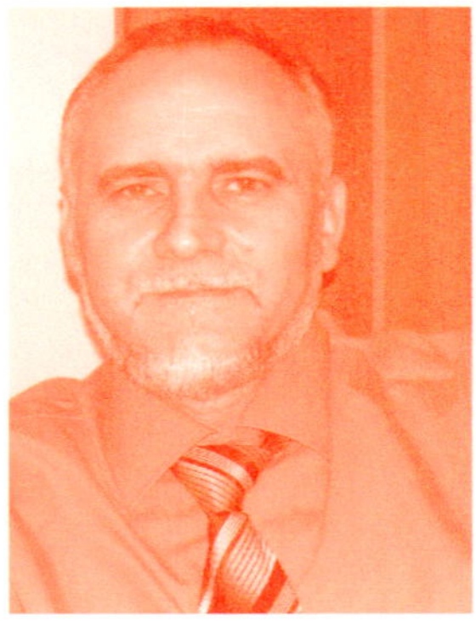
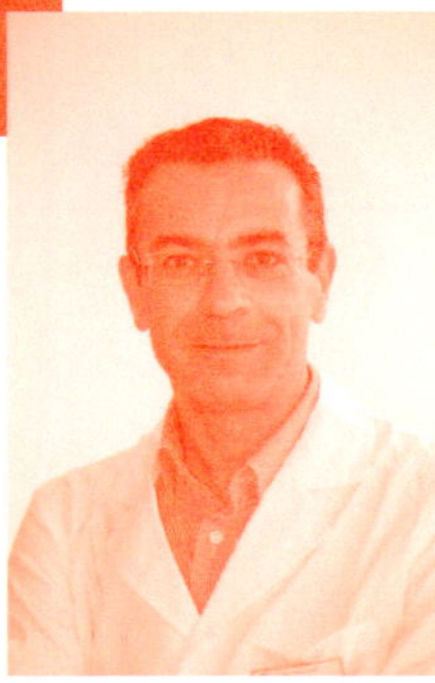
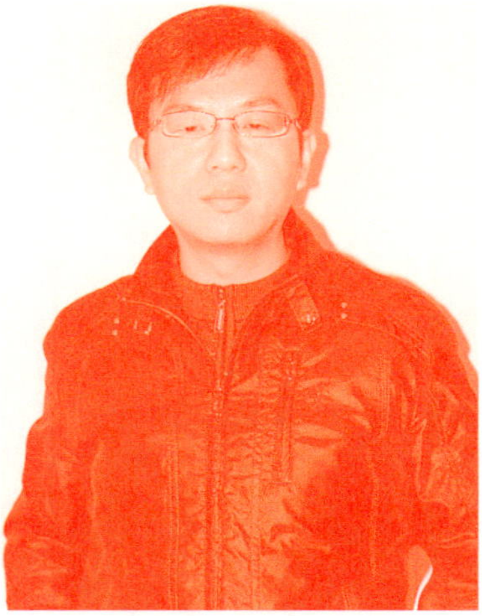
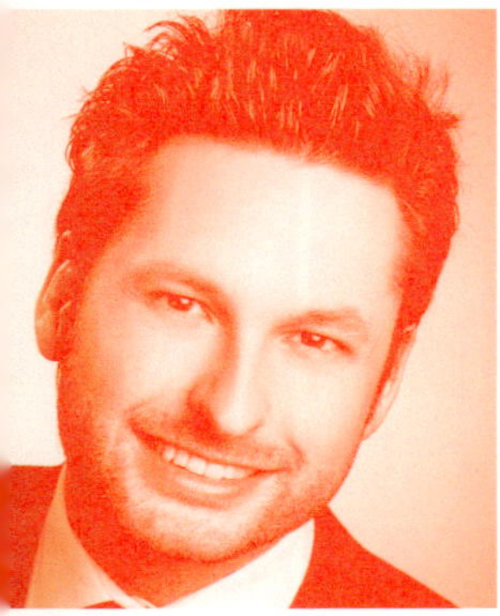
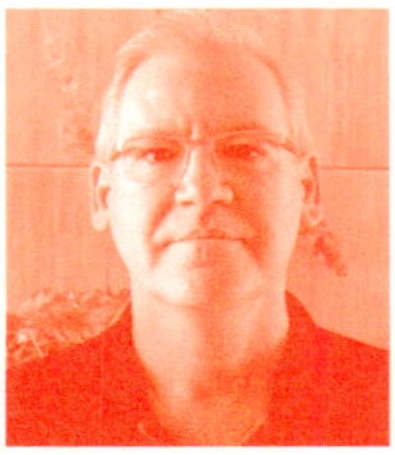

IntechOpen

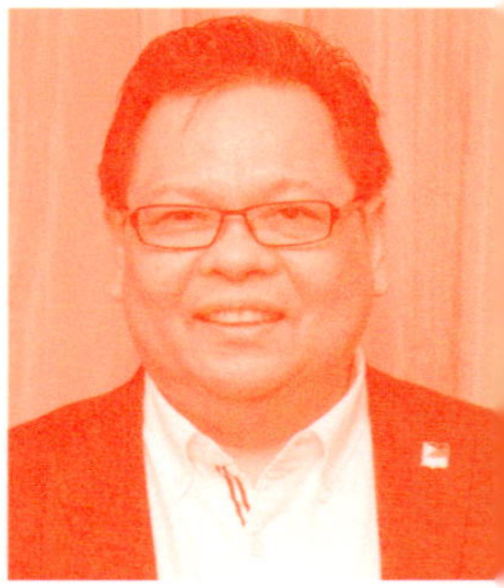
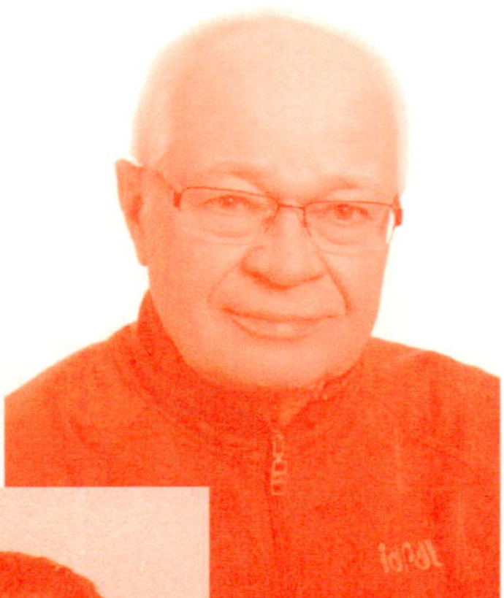
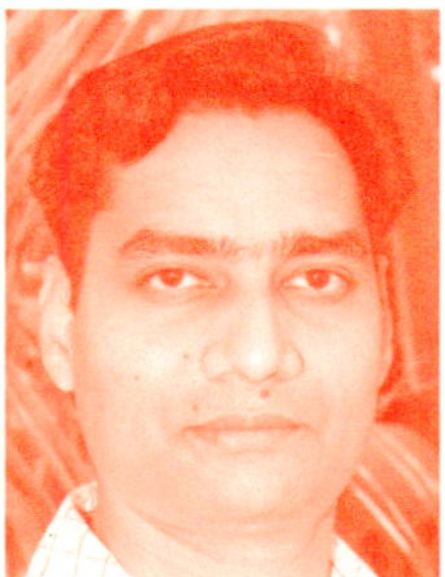
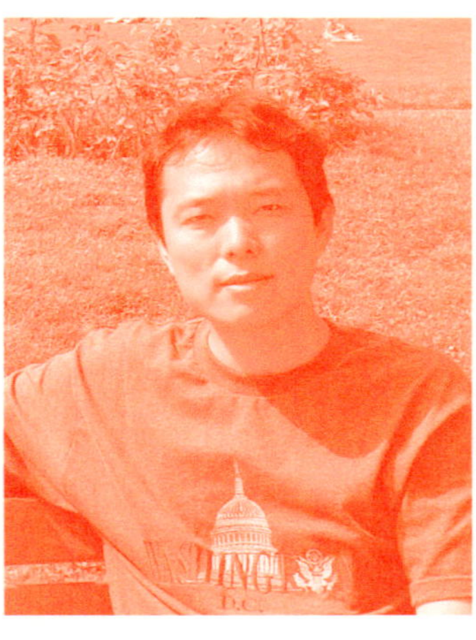
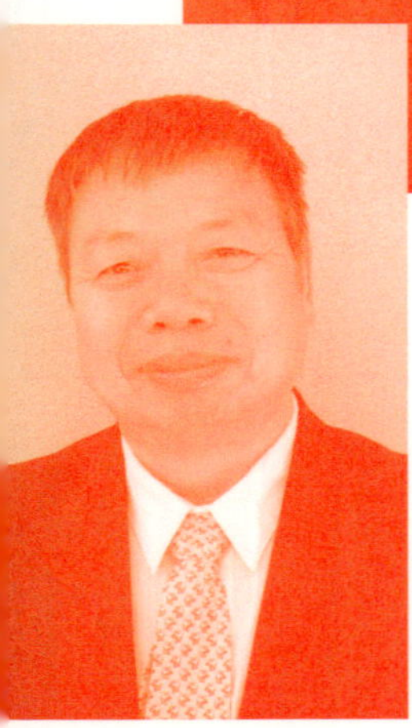
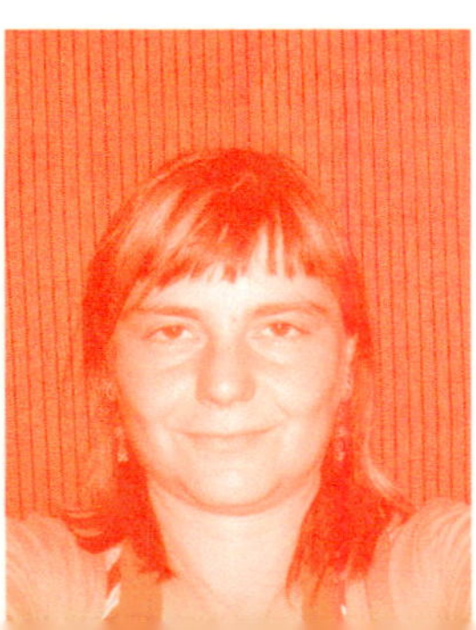

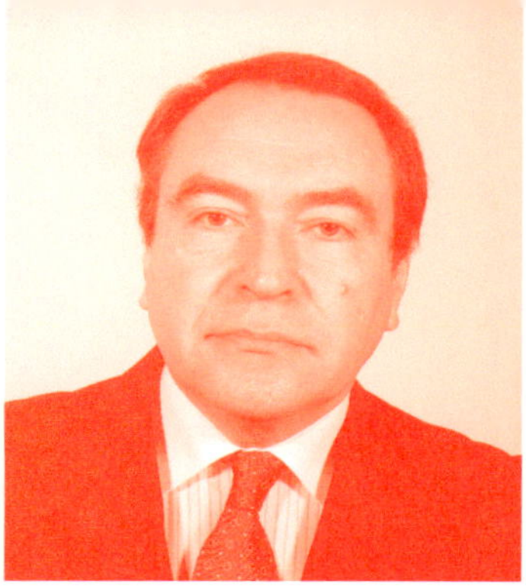
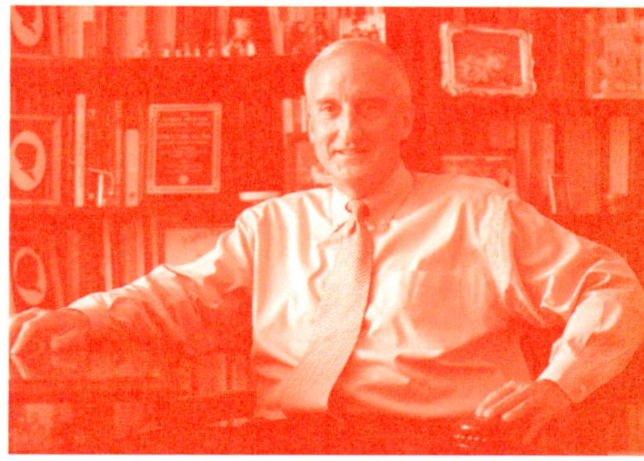
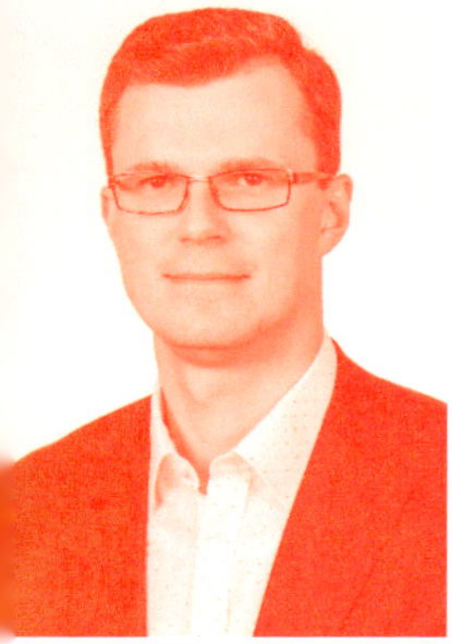
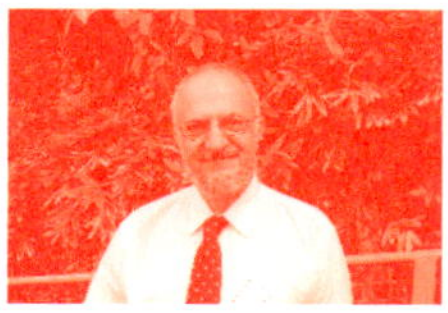
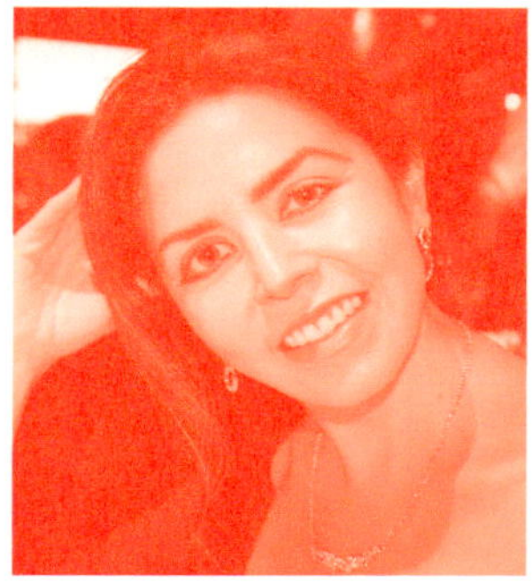

Supporting open minds since 2005

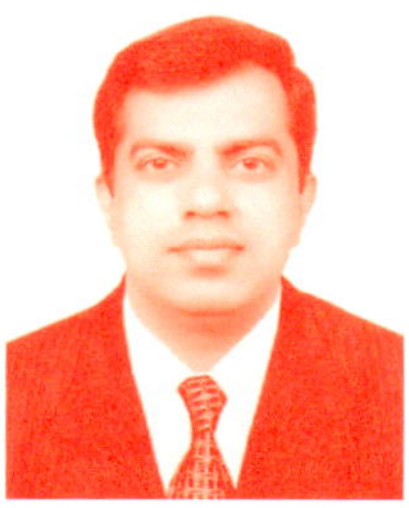
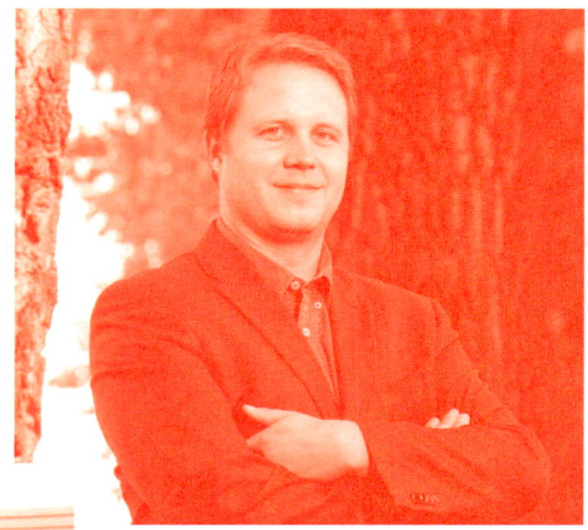
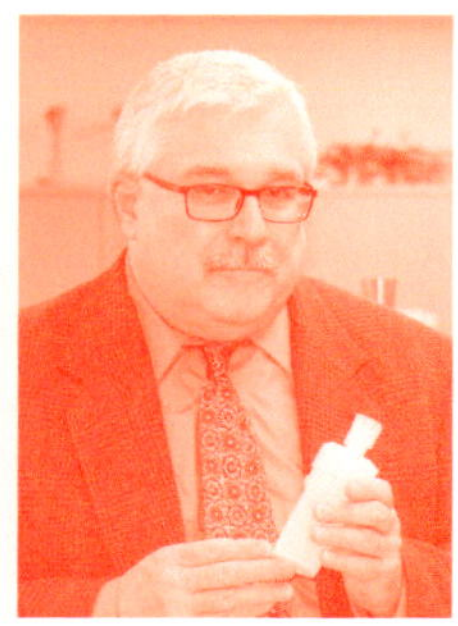
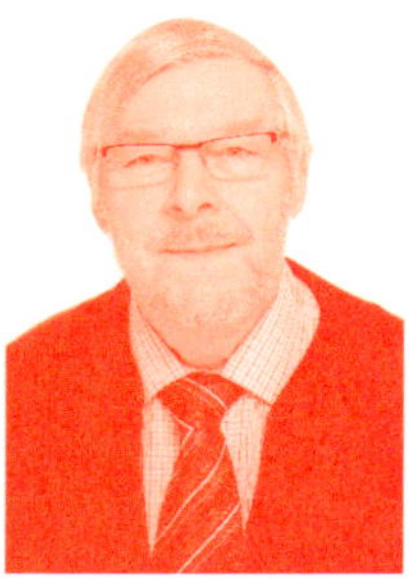
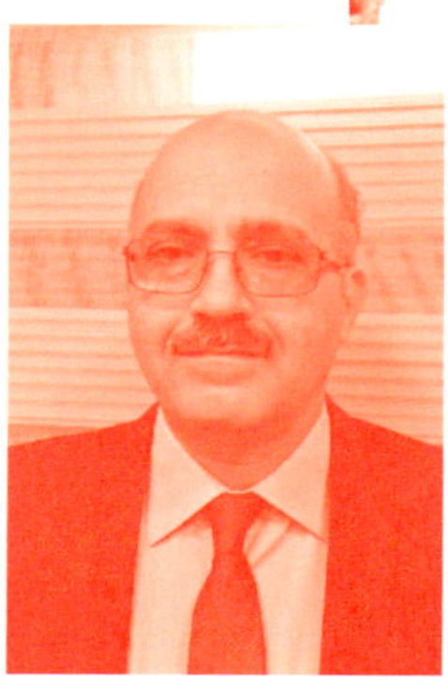
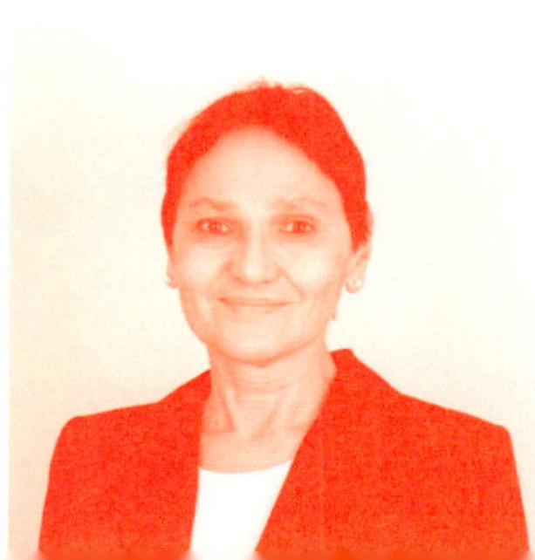
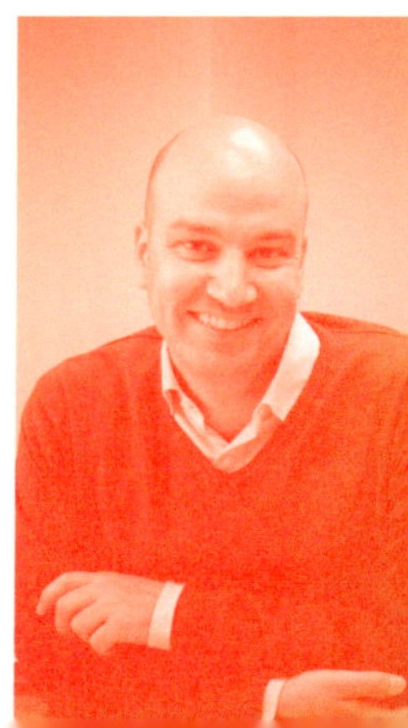

Reproductive Biology and Technology in Animals
http://dx.doi.org/10.5772/intechopen.78834
Edited by Juan Carlos Gardón Poggi and Katy Satué Ambrojo

Part of IntechOpen Book Series: Veterinary Medicine and Science, Volume 4
Book Series Editor: Rita Payan-Carreira

Contributors
Monica Cassel, Muhammad Ali, Arbab Sikandar, Verónica Mitsui Saito-Quezada, Isaías Hazarmabeth Salgado-Ugarte, Esther Uría-Galicia, José Luis Gómez-Márquez, Ana Bertha Villaseñor-Martínez, Ma. De Lourdes Jiménez-Badillo, Masahiro Sato, Kazuchika Miyoshi, Hiroaki Kawaguchi, Akihide Tanimoto, Emi Inada, Issei Saitoh, Francois Richard, Sedigheh Menatian, Jefferson Diniz, Euni Oba, Rodolpho Satrapa, Marcos Luckner, Rosano De Freitas, Rafael Satrapa, Laine Oliveira Da Silva, Marina Bento Nogueira

First published in London, United Kingdom, 2020 by IntechOpen
IntechOpen is the global imprint of INTECHOPEN LIMITED, registered in England and Wales, registration number: 11086078, 7th floor, 10 Lower Thames Street, London, EC3R 6AF, United Kingdom
Printed in Croatia

British Library Cataloguing-in-Publication Data
A catalogue record for this book is available from the British Library

Additional hard and PDF copies can be obtained from orders@intechopen.com

Reproductive Biology and Technology in Animals
Edited by Juan Carlos Gardón Poggi and Katy Satué Ambrojo
p. cm.
Print ISBN 978-1-78984-179-4
Online ISBN 978-1-78984-180-0
eBook (PDF) ISBN 978-1-78984-206-7
ISSN 2632-0517

For EU product safety concerns:
IN TECH d.o.o., Prolaz Marije Krucifikse Kozulić 3, 51000 Rijeka, Croatia, info@intechopen.com or visit our website at intechopen.com.

IntechOpen Book Series

Veterinary Medicine and Science

Volume 4

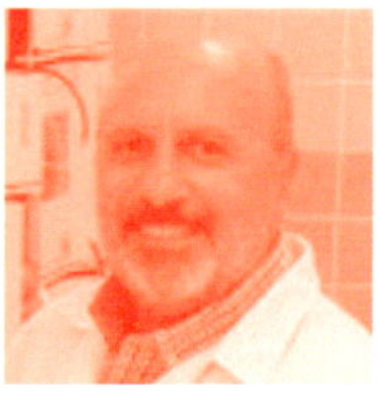

Juan Carlos Gardón Poggi received his university degree in Argentina in 1983, and his master's and PhD degrees at Córdoba University, Spain. He is currently working as a professor of the Department of Animal Medicine and Surgery at the Faculty of Veterinary and Experimental Sciences of the Catholic University of Valencia San Vicente Mártir, Valencia, Spain. He also participates in academic postgraduate activities at the Veterinary Faculty of Murcia University, Spain. He has more than 30 years of teaching and research experience. He is the author of eight book chapters and has published around 200 research papers in national and international journals and conference proceedings. He has participated as principal researcher in 12 R&D projects and the organization of seven national and international scientific events. His main research interests include animal physiology, biotechnology of reproduction either in males or females, the study of gametes under in vitro conditions, the use of ultrasound as a complement to physiological studies, and the development of reproductive applied biotechnologies. He regularly supervises students in preparing their P.D and master's theses or in final degree projects.

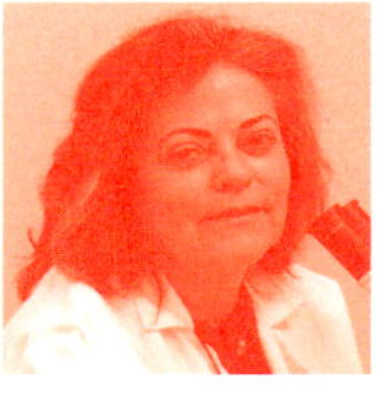

Katy Satué Ambrojo, PhD, is a professor in the Department of Animal Medicine and Surgery at the Faculty of Veterinary Medicine of the CEU-Cardenal Herrera University, Valencia, Spain. She teaches courses in general pathology, integrated in the module of applied bases of the equine veterinary clinic for the 2nd, 3rd, and 4th years of the degree program in veterinary sciences. Her research activity is focused on the fielvd of hematology, biochemistry, immunology, and fundamentally in equine endocrinology in pregnant Spanish purebreed mares. Dr. Satué has directed five PhD theses and five Certificates of Advanced Studies, has participated in 10 research projects as a collaborating researcher, and has written two books and 14 book chapters published by international publishing houses related to her research areas. She has written 70 scientific publications in international journals and has attended 70 international congresses, participating in more than 125 communications. She is also a scientific reviewer for several indexed international journals (*American Journal of Obstetrics and Gynecology*, *Journal of Equine Veterinary Science*, *Veterinary Radiology & Ultrasound*, and others). Since 2014, she has been responsible for the Clinical Analysis Laboratory of the Veterinary Clinical Hospital of CEU Cardinal Herrera University. She has also been an honorary member of the Peloritan Academy of Pericolanti since February 2018.

Editors of Volume 4: Juan Carlos Gardón Poggi
Department of Animal Medicine and Surgery
University Catholic of Valencia "San Vicente Mártir"

Katy Satué Ambrojo
Department of Animal Medicine and Surgery, Faculty of Veterinary
University of CEU-Cardenal Herrera

Book Series Editor: Rita Payan-Carreira
University of Évora, Portugal

Scope of the Series

Paralleling similar advances in the medical field, astounding advances occurred in the Veterinary Medicine and Science in recent decades, fostering a better support to animal health and more humane animal production, a better understanding of the physiology of endangered species, to improve the assisted reproductive technologies or the pathogenesis of certain diseases, where animals can be used as models for human diseases (like cancer, degenerative diseases or fertility), and even as a guarantee of public health. Bridging the Human, Animal and Environmental health, the holistic and integrative "One Health" concept intimately associates the developments within those fields, projecting its advancements into practice.
This book series aims to tackle a variety of fields in the animal-related medicine and sciences, providing thematic volumes, high quality and significance in the field, directed to researchers and postgraduates. It aims to give us a glimpse into the new accomplishments in the Veterinary Medicine and Science field. By addressing hot topics in veterinary sciences, we aim to gather authoritative texts within each issue of this series, providing in-depth overviews and analysis for graduates, academics and practitioners and foreseeing a deeper understanding of the subject. Forthcoming texts, written and edited by experienced researchers from both industry and academia, will also discuss scientific challenges faced today in Veterinary Medicine and Science. In brief, we hope that books in this series will provide accessible references for those interested or working in this field and encourage learning in a range of different topics.

Contents

Preface

We are pleased to present our new book *Reproductive Biology and Technology in Animals*. This book has been designed to provide innovative information on new reproductive technologies in different animal species, including sheep, gilts, pigs, and other invertebrates. It is intended for academics, scientists, and veterinarians to update and deepen their knowledge of the physiology of reproduction. Therefore, the motivation to publish a comprehensive volume on advances in biotechnology arose from the growing awareness of recent advances in sperm management, oocyte characteristics, various genomic aspects related to somatic cell nuclear transfer, and the microarchitecture of the female reproductive system in these animal species. Other aspects have also been considered that refer to the reproductive cycles present in gastropods and fish. This volume is the culmination of the efforts of several researchers, scientists, and scholars from around the world who are well known and respected in the various frontiers of research into the physiology of reproduction. We sincerely believe that the book will prove to be a useful contribution not only to science but also to the general public. We hope that this book will be a useful source of information from both a scientific and practical point of view. We are grateful to all the contributing authors and to all the members of the international review panel who helped us enormously with their contributions, time, critical thinking, and suggestions in producing this edited and peer-reviewed volume. The editors are also grateful to IntechOpen and its team members for the opportunity to publish this book. Finally, we thank our family members for their love, support, encouragement, and patience throughout the period of this work.

Juan Carlos Gardon Poggi
Department of Animal Medicine and Surgery,
University Catholic of Valencia "San Vicente Mártir",
Valencia, Spain

Katy Satué Ambrojo
Faculty of Veterinary,
Department of Animal Medicine and Surgery,
University of CEU-Cardenal Herrera,
Valencia, Spain

Section 1

Mammals

Chapter 1

Micro-architecture of the Female Reproductive System

Arbab Sikandar and Muhammad Ali

Abstract

The female reproductive system consists of the ovary, oviduct, uterus, and vagina. This chapter will discuss how these organs look like under the microscope and what types of ultrastructural tissues are present in it, how the shape and physiology of the tissues/cells change with the physiological activities including reproductive cycles, what type of alterations occurs in the ovary during ovulation and how its follicle and epithelium differ, and how the ovulation takes place. The chapter will also elaborate how the lining epithelium and the tract mucosa facilitate the fertilized ovum and conceptus. Also, the chapter is highlighting the architectural changes within the mucosa of the uterus during and after pregnancy and type of ovary and spermatozoa that is most suitable for fertilization.

Keywords: ovary, reproduction, microstructures, cortex, mucosa, zygote, sperm

1. Introduction

It is important to know the microstructure of the female reproductive system. In this chapter those microarchitectures are highlighted which played an important role in theriogenology right from release to fertilization and care of embryo and infants. The micro-architecture of the ovarian cortex, the microscopic structures of the follicles especially the graafian follicle including mature ova, and the histomorphology of the fimbriae and oviduct and its function in ova transportation, zygote transformation, and embryo implantation were highlighted. The microstructures of various microscopic layers of the uterus and its role in reproduction were addressed. The structure and function of the cervix and vulva and its role in reproduction are mentioned. Also, the most suitable type of ova and sperm for fertilization was also mentioned. The whole reproductive system is concerned with the production and transport of the ovum, facilitation in the transport of spermatozoa, the fusion of both gametes, and the accommodation of the embryo and fetus until birth [1].

2. Microstructure of cortex of the ovary

The cortex is a wide peripheral part of the ovary that contains follicles in various stages [2]. The surface of the ovary is covered by a thin layer of cuboidal cells, also called as germinal epithelium. Next to the germinal epithelium in the inferior side is a thick layer of connective tissue (CT) called the tunica albuginea. And the remaining portion of the ovarian cortex is covered by the CT which contains the primordial follicles, surrounded by a flat follicular cell (squamous shaped). Another follicle a bit larger is called a primary follicle, internally lined by the simple and stratified cuboidal epithelium termed as granulosa cells. In the connective tissue of the cortex of the ovary, many blood vessels surround the developing follicles. The granulosa cells are more prominent in the larger follicle called as secondary follicle or also called as antral follicle [3]. The antrum is the cavity formation within the follicle, which splits the granulosa cells into two layers. The fluid within the antrum is called as liquor folliculi. A single large ovum is present in the follicle, and a single layer of granulosa cells which surrounds the oocyte is known as corona radiata [4]. There are acellular glycoprotein layers known as zona pellucida between the corona radiata and oocyte. The zona pellucida which is 3–5 μm in thickness is produced by the ova and the granulosa cells. Within the antrum the ova are anchored by a compact mass of cells called as cumulus oophorus. After releasing the ova, the granulosa cells are disorganized within the antrum with pyknotic nuclei (fragmentation of nuclei) in the remaining follicles. This condition of the inactive follicles is called as atretic follicle [5].

3. Microstructure modulation in graafian follicle

A graafian follicle consists of a large cavity called antrum having fluid termed as follicular fluid. Graafian follicle is also known as antral follicle [3]. Before ovulation, secondary follicle undergoes first mitotic division, and as a result the graafian follicle is formed which has two N haploid chromosomes. The characteristic structural feature of graafian follicle is follicular antrum in which granulosa cell and oocyte are present. Antral follicle is a three-dimensional structure having a cavity (antrum) which is surrounded by different types of cells [6]. The antral follicle has six different histologic components which are as follows:

- The theca externa
- The theca interna
- The basal lamina
- The granulosa cell
- The oocyte
- The follicular fluid

3.1 Theca externa

Theca externa consists of smooth muscle cells that are innervated by the autonomic nerve. The functional importance of theca externa is still unclear, but there is evidence that changes in the contractile activity of theca externa are involved in atresia and ovulation [5].

3.2 Theca interna

It is consisting of different cells which are present in the matrix of loose connective tissues and blood vessels. The function of theca interna cells is regulated by luteinizing hormone (LH). Theca interna is highly vascularized, and its function is to deliver hormone, nutrients, vitamins, and cofactors, which are necessary for growth of the oocyte and granulosa cells [4].

3.3 Granulosa cells and oocyte

In the graafian follicle, the granulosa cells and oocyte have a specific shape and position [6]. There are four different types of granulosa cell layers:

- The outermost is membrana granulosa.
- The inner most is periantral.
- The intermediate is cumulus oophorus.
- Just opposed to oocyte is corona radiata.

3.4 Follicular fluid

It is rich in hyaluronan and proteoglycans. It helps in follicle ruptures. Ovulation occurs under the influence of follicle-stimulating hormone (FSH) and LH [7]. During ovulation the ova are in the metaphase stage of the second meiotic division.

4. Microstructure and physiology of the oviduct and how it facilitates the sperm, ovum, and early-stage embryo

4.1 Microstructure of the oviduct

The oviduct has several layers including the mucosa, muscular layer, and a connective serosa. The size of these layers depends on different regions of the oviduct. The myosalpinx is comprised of smooth muscle; it is thin in the region of the ampulla and multilayered thick in the region of the isthmus. The endosalpinx is a term used for a mucosa, which is lined with simple columnar ciliated epithelium [8]. In the ampulla, the lining ciliated cells are numerous compared with that of secretory cells. The lining mucosa forms folds upward that fill the tubular lumen [9]. Due to the abundance of upward-directed folds, the lining mucosa of the ampulla increased the surface area, assuming excessive ability for the metabolic conversation between the epithelial, luminal, and the underlining vascular compartments. The mucosa of the isthmus has a smaller number of folds, while the abundant number of secretory cells is present there.

4.2 Function of the oviduct

Sperm and oocyte will not reach the oviduct at the same time. In some animals the oocyte reaches first, and, in some, sperm approaches initially to the site of fertilization. The movement of sperm toward the isthmus is promoted by the ciliary movement of the lining epithelium. The spermatozoa are stored and remain active in the oviduct for up to 72 hours, but in some species the time is extended for a month like in bats. The fallopian tube contains fluid secreted by the glandular epithelium, which has a positive impact on the viability of sperm and provides nutrition to the oocyte [8]. This fluid helps in the maturation of the oocyte in the oviduct. Sperm adhere to the epithelial wall of the fallopian tube which preserves its viability and stops the premature capacitation. This enhances the chances of fertilization [1].

Fertilization of the ovum results in the formation of zygotes. After all the embryonic changes in the zygote, the later embryo is transferred along the fallopian tube. Some hormone also helps in the transportation of the embryo. The production of the estradiol (E2) by the embryo also helps in its transportation. In the mare, the secretion of prostaglandin (PGE2) during the first week acts on the oviduct locally and causes the transfer of the embryo to the posterior region of the uterus. The 4- to 8-cell stage embryos in hamster secrete platelet-activating factor (PAF). The later factor also acts on the oviduct locally, resulting in the transfer of the embryo toward the uterine horns. It is important to note that in the hamster and the mare, the main factor, decisive whether and when the fertilized ovum will drive toward the uterine horns or not, is based on the condition of the fertilized eggs.

4.3 Transportation of oocyte

During ovulation the fimbriae attached to the surface of graafian follicle and sweep the ova further anterior toward the ampulla [8]. The coordinated contraction of the myosalpinx along the length of the fallopian tube and the ciliary beats of the epithelial cells results in the transportation of the oocyte to the site of fertilization [9].

5. Microstructures and physiology of fimbriae

Fimbriae are finger-like growth processes that are present at the terminal of each fallopian tube. They increase the surface area of the infundibulum and cause it to slip over the surface of the ovary when ovulation occurs. This activity of the fimbriae increases the possibility that the oozed-out oocyte will be captured after ovulation from the graafian follicle and transported through a wider opening called ostium into the ampulla of the oviduct [9]. Above the mucus membrane of the fallopian tube, there are three layers of tissues, viz., the innermost layer consists of spirally arranged fibers, the middle layer consists of fibers with circular arrangement, and the outermost sheath has longitudinally arranged fibers that end in fimbriae near ovaries, forming a funnel-shaped depository structure called the infundibulum. One fimbria out of all fimbriae is long enough to reach the external surface of the ovary, which is called as fimbria ovarica [10]. The fallopian tube at this point is lined by small epithelial cells with small, slender hair-like cilia pulsating unidirectionally inside the fallopian tube to guide and direct the ovum from the ovary to the uterus [9].

5.1 Role of fimbriae in directing the ova to area of fertilization

As there is no direct connection between ovaries and the oviduct, the egg is transported to the uterus in peritoneal fluid produced by fimbriae on the terminal of tube's opening. The specialized granulosa cells of oocyte (cumulus oophorous) at ovulation are sticky and help in adhering to the surface of fimbriae. After this the fimbriae through muscular control create negative pressure that picks up oocyte and moves it to the fallopian tube [9]. There are also some hormonal changes that control the picking up of oocyte [7].

5.2 Process of fertilization within the fallopian tube

At the site of ampulla-isthmus junction, the capacitated and hyperactive spermatozoa crossed the layer of corona radiata and pierced the glycoprotein layer of zona pellucida. Afterward the fusion of the spermatozoa with the ova takes place [11], which results in the formation of zygote.

6. Histological layers, physiology of the uterus, and its role in reproduction

If we see the cross section of the uterus, it consists of four layers including the innermost mucosa, the submucosa, the muscularis, and the outermost serosa [9].

6.1 Mucosa

It is the innermost layer facing the lumen. It is lined with secretary layers of columnar epithelium. The embryo after a series of changes including zygote, two-cell (blastomeres) stage, morula (16-cell stage), blastula (inner cell mass leads to embryo, and the outer cell mass leads to the formation of the placenta, with the formation of fluid filled cavity), and gastrula (where formation of three characteristic embryonic germ layers occurs) is implanted in the endometrial mucosa with a layer of trophoblast [1]. The trophoblastic cell layers are proliferated in the lamina propria (uterine stroma) forming lacunae. The lacunae form an open connection with the maternal sinusoid in the uterine stroma, which results in the establishment of the uteroplacental circulation. The endometrial glands develop from the mucosa and invaginate inward into the submucosa adopting a coiled shape. The endometrial glands secrete PGF2 alpha at a critical time during estrous cycle that causes luteolysis of corpus luteum if the animal is not pregnant [12]. The endometrium of ruminants has caruncles that are highly vascularized and provide a maternal portion of the placenta if attachment of the embryo occurs. While these caruncles are absent in sow and mare, instead endometrial folds are present. These endometrial folds provide uterine surface for the attachment of the placenta. So, the uterus is the place where attachment and nourishment of the fertilized ova take place, and it helps in pushing the baby during parturition [8].

6.2 Submucosa

After the mucosa, a layer of submucosa is present. It houses a rich blood supply, nerve endings, and the lymphatics in addition to the rich supply of mononuclear cells. It has a role in providing nutrition and maintaining coordination and has supporting effect to the mucosa [9]. The muscularis is present beneath the submucosa and consists of double arranged layers of smooth muscles like longitudinal muscles (outer layer) and inner circular muscles (inner layer). A very prominent third layer of smooth muscle in oblique arrangement can also be seen in the gravid uterus. These layers played a very important function by providing the uterus with the ability to contract, and that contraction is very important on the following basis:

- Transportation of the secretary products
- Transportation of the gametes (sperm and ova)

- Movement of early embryo to the appropriate location
- Maintaining and nourishment of the embryo and fetus

It also has a key role in the expulsion of the fetus and fetal membranes at the time of parturition.

6.3 Serosa

It is the outer covering of the uterus that consists of a single layer of squamous cells.

7. Gross and microscopic structures and functions of the cervix

The whole reproductive tract is tubular except the ovary. The cervix is a thick-walled tubular structure where mucosa-submucosa-derived folds or rings are present, but their number varies from species to species. Only onefold is seen in bitch and queen, but multiple folds are seen in cow, ewe, sow, and mare. In cow and ewe, rings/folds are having interlocking finger-like projections. In pigs, rings interdigitate so interdigitation is seen in them. The cervix is soft in mare due to the presence of loose folds of the mucosa. In a bitch the cervix is smooth due to lack of folds. The primary function of the cervix is lubrication of the canal which is required during copulation [8]. Lubrication is by two types of secretions, e.g., the sulfomucin which is viscous (mobility is directed toward exterior (vagina) and inhibits sperm transport in the uterus), and the sialomucins which facilitate the sperm to move into the uterus. The cervix isolates the conceptus inside the uterus from the outer environment by the formation of cervical seal under the action of progesterone which thickens the mucus produced in the cervix and glues the folding together to prevent entry of microbes during pregnancy.

Like other tubular organs, it consists of four tunics/laminae, i.e., mucosa, submucosa, muscularis, and serosa/adventitia [9]. The mucosal tunics of the endocervix are lined by simple columnar epithelium along with the presence of mucus-producing cells called goblet cells. In some animal species, a few columnar cells are found ciliated and in simple tubular glands may be seen in the ruminant's mucosa. In the case of pigs, up to 90% of the mucosal lining epithelium is stratified squamous. Most of the ectocervical portion of the cervical mucosa is lined by the stratified squamous epithelium. Mucosa and the submucosa form folds into the cervical lumen. These folds vary in height, width, and thickness from species to species. The lamina propria of the mucosa and submucosa combines to form propria-submucosa. This propria-submucosa is heavily infiltrated by dense irregular connective tissue and supply of rich blood vessels extended deep in the submucosa. The muscularis layer is composed of two smooth muscle layers. The inner layer is circular layer and the outer layer is longitudinal in arrangements. The myenteric plexus is present in the muscular layers. Some elastic fibers are also observed in this layer. Serosa/adventitia is a loose connective tissue layer present in the outer surface. This layer is surrounded by the mesothelium which is a layer of simple squamous epithelium. Gartner's ducts may be seen in serosal layer unilateral or bilateral.

7.1 Functions of the cervix

During estrus stage of estrous cycle, the mucosa is responsible for mucus secretion. Dense irregular connective tissue becomes edematous and forms areolar structure, i.e., loose connective tissue. Circular muscular layer along with elastic fiber is responsible for the involution of the cervix after parturition [8].

8. Gross and microscopic anatomy of the vulva and its role in reproduction

The vulva is the most outer part of the female reproductive track immediately external to the vaginae. It is composed of various structures, including the mons pubis, clitoris, labia minora, labia majora, vulvar vestibule, vestibulovaginal bulbs, urethral meatus, hymen, and Bartholin and Skene glands and ducts. Bartholin glands are like the bulbourethral glands in male. The female clitoris is like the penis of the males [13]. The hymen is the stratified squamous nonkeratinized epithelium. The lateral vulvar surfaces are made up of labia majora and are comprised of fibrous and adipose folds. The labia minora also consists of connective tissue in two folds containing few (if any) adipose tissues. The labia minora is bifurcated anteriorly. The vestibule is the zone between Hart's line and the hymen, which consists of stratified squamous nonkeratinized epithelium [9]. The following are the glands present in the vulvar region of the female reproductive system:

- Apocrine glands (scent glands)
- Skene glands
- Sebaceous glands
- Eccrine glands (sweat glands)

8.1 Microscopic anatomy of vulva

Vaginal lining epithelium is stratified squamous and nonkeratinized, whereas the epithelium of the labia majora is stratified squamous and keratinized. Microscopic layers of the vulva are the mucosa, submucosa, muscularis, and serosa [14, 15]. Glands are present in the submucosal layer and the innermost layer is the mucosa.

8.2 Role of the vulva in reproduction

Being a gateway to the uterus, its primary role is to offer protection by closing the labia [16]. The external uterine orifice is protected by the vulva supported by thick large lips of labia majora along with small lips of labia minora. The urethra also opens in the vulva that is known as the urethral meatus, thus performing a function of urine passage. It also gives the pathway for sperm for entry in the body. Sometimes due to the folds and the moisture, the fungal infection may occur. The area between the opening of the vagina and the anus, below the labia majora, is called the perineum [12]. By observing the vulva, we can detect if the female is in estrous or not. If the vulva is thick and edematous, it is in the heat, and if not the female is not in the heat; this is due to the estrogen level in the female body. The penis like clitoris detects the nerve stimuli and performs the following functions:

- Enabling sperm to enter in the body of female
- Protecting the internal genital organs from infection causing organisms
- Providing the sexual pleasure

9. Type of sperm which is most favorable for fertilization

As we know around 250 million sperm cells enter the female external genitalia, but just a few thousands can enter the fallopian tube, and only a single sperm will fertilize the ova [14]. Several problems and barriers came in the pathway of the spermatozoa to touch the final goal. These range from the low pH in and around the vagina, the mucus of the cervix, the narrowness of the uterotubal junction (the entrance of the cervix), the WBCs of the immune system which treat the spermatozoa as a foreign entity to destroy, cell-to-cell interactions, gene expression, phenotypic sperm traits, sperm motility defects, DNA status, lack of capacitation or morphological normality, and failure of abnormal spermatozoa to reach to the site of fertilization. The wall of seminiferous tubules which are the coiled structure is responsible to produce the sperm. For a spermatozoon, around 28–42 days is lapsed to cross the male reproductive system. In the female reproductive tract, sperm undergo changes that help in fertilization called activation and capacitation, but all sperm are not capacitated at the same time; therefore, all sperm are not able to fertilize the cells [16]. However, several mechanisms that aid this process are good motility, adequate morphology, and normal DNA status of the cell. A sperm which has normal head, nucleus, and tail and has a moderate motility is considerable to fertilize the egg [17]. The sperm are guided upon their journey by the chemical and the temperature signals. A sperm reservoir in the fallopian tubes, where sperms bind to the epithelial lining (columnar in shape) of the tubes, reduces the chance of fertilization by multiple sperm. During ovulation, the sperm are hyperactivated to help them to the penetration of the mucus in the fallopian tubes and the outer coating of the egg. Sperm outer membrane fuses with egg outer membrane to facilitate fertilization. Acrosomal reaction occurs in the sperm head once the spermatozoa reached the ova. Acrosin enzyme helps in acrosomal reaction. Hyaluronic acid enzyme has an important role in the permeability and motility of sperms and their interactions with gametes. Formation of a functional reservoir through epithelial binding of sperm to the oviductal isthmus reduces the likelihood of the polyspermic fertilization. Motility or hyperactivation helps sperm in penetrating the mucus in the fallopian tubes and the cumulus oophorus (corona radiata), and the acrosome exocytosis may assist penetration of oocyte zona pellucida that proceeds the fusion within oocyte plasma membrane. Zona pellucida then undergoes biochemical changes so that further sperm cannot penetrate the cell called zona block [17]. In addition to alteration of zona pellucida, the cortical reaction reduces the ability of oocyte plasma membrane to fuse with additional spermatozoa, thus causing vitelline block. Both zona block and vitelline block prevent polyspermy.

10. The type of ova that is most favorable for fertilization

Fertilization is a process in which male and female gametes fuse to form a zygote. Ovum is the female gamete, and its selection is the criteria of fertilization. There are many factors that are responsible for its selection including follicular dominance, cumulus oophorus formation, cumulus oocyte complex formation, fimbrial supportive structure, and zona pellucidal layer that enable sperm to fuse with ovum.

Follicular dominance is based on E2 production. The follicle, which has greater ability of E2 production, has greater capability of its dominance. Dominancy is responsible for onward ovulation. Ovulated egg is surrounded by two protective layers [9]. Corona radiata is the outermost layer containing granulosal cells, and zona pellucida is the innermost thick transparent glycoprotein membranes surrounding the plasma membranes. With a maturation of oocyte, multiple granulosal cells enlarge called cumulus oophorus [3]. This oocyte and granulosal cells form complex known as cumulus oocyte complex (COC). The cumulus of mature COC adheres to the surface of fimbriae as sticky substances. After the sex hormones signal the fimbriae, it contracts and releases oocyte. After release, oocyte has only 24–28 hours to fuse with sperm; otherwise, it is lost. Oocyte releases some chemicals that attract the sperm, and the sperm tries to penetrate two protective layers of oocyte. First it burrows to the cell of corona radiata and then move toward zona pellucida layer. Zona pellucida is composed of four glycoproteins ZP1, ZP2, ZP3, and ZP4. The primary ligand of sperm oocyte binding is ZP3 and ZP4. Both induce acrosomal reaction of sperm to complete fusion reaction and form a zygote [18]. These factors make the ovum gamete most favorable for fertilization.

11. Conclusion

The microarchitectural examination of the reproductive organs at microscopic level is very much important to recognize its structure and function during reproductive physiology. Furthermore, this chapter highlighted the dealing of the lining mucosa with the fertilized ovum and conceptus.

Acknowledgements

The author would like to acknowledge the efforts of Prof. Dr. Ashiq Hussain Cheema for facilitating and guiding. Furthermore, Jr. lab attendant Mr. Saqib Ali, is hereby acknowledged in helping me in the write-up.

Author details

Arbab Sikandar[1]* and Muhammad Ali[2]

1 Sub-campus, Jhang, University of Veterinary and Animal Sciences, Lahore, Pakistan

2 University College of Veterinary and Animal Sciences, The Islamia University of Bahawalpur, Pakistan

*Address all correspondence to: drarbab786@gmail.com; arbab.sikandar@uvas.edu.pk

References

[1] Arrotéia KF, Garcia PV, Barbieri MF, Justino ML, Pereira LAV. The epididymis: Embryology, structure, function and its role in fertilization and infertility. In: Pereira LAV, ed. Embryology-Updates and Highlights on Classic Topics. Rijeka, Croatia: IntechOpen; 2012. DOI: 10.5772/2142

[2] Osvaldo-Decima L. Smooth muscle in the ovary of the rat and monkey. Journal of Ultrastructure Research. 1970;**30** (1–2):218-237

[3] Fortune JE. Ovarian follicular growth and development in mammals. Biology of Reproduction. 1994;**50**(2):225-232

[4] Hyttel PFTCH, Fair T, Callesen H, Greve T. Oocyte growth, capacitation and final maturation in cattle. Theriogenology. 1997;**47**(1):23-32

[5] Saidapur SK. Follicular atresia in the ovaries of nonmammalian vertebrates. In: International Review of Cytology. Vol. 54. New York: Academic Press; 1978. pp. 225-244

[6] Rodgers RJ, Irving-Rodgers HF. Morphological classification of bovine ovarian follicles. Reproduction. 2010; **139**(2):309

[7] Wiley C, Jahnke M, Redifer C, Gunn PJ, Dohlman T. Effects of endogenous progesterone during ovarian follicle superstimulation on embryo quality and quantity in beef cows. Theriogenology. 2019;**129**:54-60

[8] Padubidri VG, Daftary SN, editors. Shaw's Textbook of Gynecology-EBOOK. Elsevier, India: Elsevier Health Sciences; 2018

[9] Boyd KL, Muehlenbachs A, Rendi MH, Garcia RL, Gibson-Corley KN. Female reproductive system. In: Comparative Anatomy and Histology. London, United Kingdom: Academic Press; 2018. pp. 303-334

[10] Guan J, Watrelot A. Fallopian subtle pathology. Best Practice and Research Clinical Obstetrics and Gynaecology. 2019. https://doi.org/10.1016/j.bpobgyn.2018.12.012

[11] Carlson BM. Human Embryology and Developmental Biology E-Book. New York: Elsevier Health Sciences; 2018

[12] Bazer FW, Burghardt RC, Johnson GA, Spencer TE, Wu G. Mechanisms for the establishment and maintenance of pregnancy: Synergies from scientific collaborations. Biology of Reproduction. 2018;**99**(1):225-241

[13] Baskin L, Shen J, Sinclair A, Cao M, Liu X, Liu G, et al. Development of the human penis and clitoris. Differentiation. 2018;**103**:74-85

[14] Vuarin P, Hingrat Y, Lesobre L, Jalme MS, Lacroix F, Sorci G. Sperm competition accentuates selection on ejaculate attributes. Biology Letters. 2019;**15**(3):20180889

[15] Kumar V. Histological, histochemical and scanning electron microscopic studies on the oviduct and uterus of jaffarabadi buffalo (*Bubalus bubalis*) during follicular and luteal phases 2514 (doctoral dissertation). Junagadh: JAU; 2018

[16] Lucas D, Fox J. The psychology of human sexuality. The psychology of human sexuality. In: Noba Textbook Series: Psychology. Champaign, IL: DEF Publishers; 2018

[17] Lehmann R. Matchmaking molecule for egg and sperm. Science. 2018; **361**(6406):974-975

[18] Hirohashi N, Yanagimachi R. Sperm acrosome reaction: Its site and role in fertilization. Biology of Reproduction. 2018

Chapter 2

Oocyte Meiotic Resumption under High Surveillance

François J. Richard

Abstract

Germinal vesicle breakdown (GVBD) is the hallmark of oocyte meiotic resumption. It occurs under minimal stimulation during in vitro maturation (IVM). Several factors have been described to be involved in the inhibition of oocyte meiotic resumption such as purine derivatives. This study was assessing whether adenosinergic and guanosinergic systems are functional and participating in the inhibition of oocyte maturation. The objectives of the present study were to evaluate the effect of two purines, adenosine (ADO) and guanosine (GUO), on in vitro oocyte meiotic resumption, cumulus cell expansion, and gap junction communication. Both ADO and GUO significantly inhibited GVBD oocytes. The inhibitory effect lasted 24 hours and was reversible for meiotic resumption and cumulus cell expansion. Both ADO and GUO increased gap junction communication in cumulus cells. Equine chorionic gonadotropin (eCG) and the adenylyl cyclase stimulator, forskolin (FK), were both supportive of ADO and GUO inhibitory effect. The results are suggesting both adenosinergic and guanosinergic systems efficient in inhibiting oocyte meiotic resumption. The use of these two systems as part of a pre-IVM culture period would be a novel strategy to explore in order to improve oocyte developmental competence.

Keywords: oocyte, purine, adenosine, guanosine, meiotic resumption

1. Introduction

Oocyte meiosis begins during fetal development in large animals such as in cow, sow, and ewe. Once the sub-phases of the first prophase are completed, the oocyte meiosis stops at the dictyate stage. At this point, crossing over is a past event and chromatin is accessible for transcription. This G2/M phase transition of the cell cycle characterizes mammalian oocytes. The female gamete bears 4n chromosomes as long as the ovulatory LH peak generates its effect on the preovulatory follicle to induce oocyte meiotic resumption. Dysregulation of the oocyte cell cycle induced by c-MOS proto-oncogene after gene null mutation caused parthenogenic development of the oocyte and explained female mouse infertility [1]. This phenotype illustrates how important it is to appropriately control oocyte meiotic resumption.

Oocyte meiotic resumption is a highly important physiological event for species survival since it refers to a successful reproduction by appropriately preparing the female gamete. This unique cell division has to occur at the right time and imply high surveillance. From an evolutionary point of view, the number of female gametes produced went from a large number, such as in frog, to a small number in mammals. Although several thousands of oocytes are found in the ovaries, only a small percentage is ovulated, and even less are fertilized. Considering this selective restriction, a framework of the meiotic resumption process has developed. Throughout the evolutionary process, mechanisms have been added to ensure a very precise control of this crucial event related to species survival, which is the final phase of gamete preparation for fertilization. Interestingly, the role of EGF-like peptides fully fits with this notion. It is well-known that the LH peak induces oocyte meiotic resumption in the preovulatory follicles. However, the EGF-like peptides are also active participants in the ovulatory process, meiotic resumption, and cumulus cell expansion, clearly supporting an add-up to the LH surge. Going back to the control of oocyte meiotic resumption, although the contribution of cAMP and cGMP is well described, it is obvious that other mechanisms may still be involved and be discovered.

It has long been known that adenosine (ADO) is a molecule playing an important role in various physiological systems such as in the central nervous system and cardiac function [2]. On the other hand, there are very few studies on the role of ADO in mammalian ovarian follicle. ADO is known to act on specific receptors, to cross plasma membrane using transporters, and to be generated from functional catabolism by extracellular enzymes, a system called adenosinergic [3]. On the other hand, guanosine (GUO) has not been as popular in research. However, in recent years a new interest on GUO has revealed its importance in the effect of ADO on the functioning of the central nervous system [4]. Although no specific receptor for GUO has been yet identified, its physiological impact leaves no doubt. GUO has neuroprotective effects, it diminishes the apoptotic effects observed in Parkinson's disease, and it also has a protective role during a challenge with glutamate, during mitochondrial stress, and during ischemia [4–6]. Because GUO can also be generated by a functional catabolism using extracellular enzymes, these results support the existence of a so-called guanosinergic system.

ADO has also been identified in the follicular fluid with several other purine derivatives. Among these derivatives, hypoxanthine is the compound that has attracted the most studies in last three decades. In mice, ADO improves the inhibitory effect of hypoxanthine on the resumption of meiosis but has no effect when used alone, even at a dose of 5 mM [7]. In the rat, the effect of ADO is also minimal [8]. In cattle, ADO used at 200 μM slowed meiotic resumption [9]. There is one study reporting that it has not been able to measure GUO in follicular fluid [10]. In contrast, GUO showed a very potent effect on the inhibition of meiotic resumption in mice [10] and rat [8].

This study is proposing to assess whether an adenosinergic and guanosinergic system are functional and participating in the inhibition of oocyte meiotic resumption. Specifically, the research presented here aims to study the involvement of ADO and GUO in the physiology of the ovarian follicle by targeting their effect on in vitro meiotic resumption using swine as the animal model.

2. Material and methods

2.1 Chemicals

Unless otherwise stated, all chemicals were purchased from Sigma Chemical Co. (St. Louis, MO, USA). The adenylyl cyclase activator, forskolin (FK), was prepared as a millimolar stock solution and stored at −20°C as already described [11]. ADO and GUO were prepared from the stock powder directly in the culture medium on the day of the experiment. 8-Bromoadenosine (8-BrADO) and 8-Bromoguanosine (8-BrGUO) were dissolved in DMSO, and a DMSO control was run simultaneously.

The chemicals were added to the maturation medium a few hours prior to the addition of the oocytes.

2.2 Ovary collections

As previously described, prepubertal gilt ovaries were collected from a local slaughterhouse [12]. In brief, they were placed in saline (0.9% NaCl containing antibiotics and antimycotics, 100,000 IU/L penicillin G, 100 mg/L streptomycin, 250 μg/L amphotericin B) and kept at 37°C. They were rinsed once in a fresh saline solution having antibiotics and antimycotics at 37°C.

2.3 Maturation medium

Oocytes were matured in BSA-free North Carolina State University 23 (NCSU) medium [13] supplemented with 25 μM β-mercaptoethanol (Bio-Rad, Hercules, CA, USA), 0.1 mg/mL cysteine, 10% (v/v) porcine follicular fluid (PFF), and gonadotropins (2.5 IU/well for hCG [APL, Ayerst Laboratories Inc., Philadelphia, PA, USA] and 2.5 IU/well for eCG [Folligon, Intervet, Whitby, ON, Canada]) [12]. PFF was collected from follicles of 2–6 mm in diameter. After centrifugation (1500×*g*, 30 minutes), the supernatant was filtered (0.8 and 0.45 μm) and stored at −20°C until used [11].

2.4 Recovery of cumulus-oocyte complexes (COC)

Cumulus-oocyte complexes were collected from follicles of 2–6 mm in diameter. They were aspirated with a 10-mL syringe and an 18G needle [11]. The follicular contents were pooled in 50-mL conical tubes (Falcon, Franklin Lakes, NJ, USA). The pellet was washed twice with HEPES-buffered Tyrode's medium containing 0.01% (w/v) polyvinyl alcohol (PVA-TLH) [14]. The COC were recovered under a stereomicroscope and transferred to a petri dish containing PVA-TLH. The COC were washed three times with PVA-TLH and then subjected to their respective treatments. Groups of 20–30 COC were placed in the wells of four-well multi-dishes (Nunc, Roskilde, Denmark) containing 500 μL of maturation medium. The COC were cultured at 38.5°C, 5% CO_2 in 95% air atmosphere with 100% humidity.

2.5 Selecting COC and denuding oocytes

The criteria of selection were COC with a minimum of three layers of clear and compact cumulus cells which surrounded the oocyte [12]. Those with dark, pyknotic, or expanded cumulus cells, and those containing oocytes with a very clear cytoplasm or of small diameter were rejected. The oocytes were denuded of their cumulus cells by drawing several times the COC into a pipette using PVA-TLH. Once denuded, the oocytes were rinsed in PVA-TLH, and those with a homogeneous cytoplasm were selected.

2.6 Assessment of oocyte nuclear maturation stage

The oocyte nuclear maturation stage was evaluated following a 48-hour fixation period in a solution of ethanol and acetic acid (3:1). Using a phase contrast microscope at 100 and 400× magnification immediately after staining with 1% aceto-orcein [15] allows us to assess oocyte nuclear maturation stage. Those having a nuclear membrane were considered at the germinal vesicle (GV) stage, whereas those without a nuclear membrane were considered to have resumed meiosis. The oocytes were considered mature when they were in anaphase I, telophase I, and metaphase II.

2.7 Cumulus-cumulus gap-FRAP assay to measure gap junction communications (GJC)

After 4 hours of in vitro culture, COC were loaded with calcein-AM (39,69-di(*O*-acetyl)-29,79-bis(*N*,*N*-bis(carboxymethyl) amino methyl)-fluorescein) and tetra(acetoxymethyl ester) (Molecular Probes C-3100) in IVM medium containing 0.1 mg/mL PVA [16]. After 20 minutes at 38.5°C, the live COC were mounted on glass slides in the PVA-containing IVM medium. Fluorescence recovery after photobleaching (FRAP) assays were conducted using Nikon Eclipse TE2000-E inverted confocal microscope. The bleaching was performed for 5 minutes using laser pulses on a limited region of cumulus cells observed at a magnification of 90×. The COC were photographed at 60× before bleaching and every 3 minutes thereafter for 12 minutes. Fluorescence intensity was quantified using ImageJ software (National Institutes of Health, USA). A relative fluorescence value was achieved by dividing the raw fluorescence measurement in the bleached area by the mean fluorescence in two adjacent regions. This value was further divided by the fluorescence value of a region at the opposite end of the COC to correct for unintended bleaching caused by the laser excitation.

2.8 Statistical analyses

All values are presented with their corresponding SEM, and the number of replicates is indicated for each experiment (at least three). The data were analyzed by one-way ANOVA using GraphPad Prism v7.02 for Windows (GraphPad Software, San Diego, CA, USA). When ANOVA indicated a significant effect of treatment ($P < 0.05$), individual treatment differences were compared using Bonferroni's multiple comparison post-hoc test. Significant effects were identified by * or different letters.

3. Results

In our hands, prior to in vitro maturation, more than 95% of swine oocytes have not started their nuclear maturation, that is, their meiotic resumption (<5% of GVDB oocytes), and cumulus cells have not expanded yet [12].

3.1 Adenosine inhibits oocyte meiotic resumption

The first experiment is aiming to assess ADO on inhibition of oocyte GVBD. When COC are cultured for 24 hours in control treatment, more than 94.3 ± 3.0% of the oocytes were in GVBD, that is, oocyte meiotic resumption took place (**Figure 1A**). The inhibitory effect of ADO was dose-dependent with only 13.9 ± 2.1% in GVBD after an exposure to ADO at 2.0 mM for 24 hours (**Figure 1A**). The EC_{50} of ADO on the percentage of GVBD oocyte is calculated as already described [11] and determined to be 1.3 mM. In addition, at 2.0 mM ADO inhibited cumulus cell expansion (**Figure 1B5**) compared with the control (**Figure 1B1**). When cultured for 24 hours as oocytes denuded of their cumulus cells (DO), ADO (2.0 mM) did not significantly inhibit oocyte GVBD compared with the control conditions (**Figure 1C**). These results support an inhibitory effect of ADO on both oocyte meiotic resumption and cumulus expansion when cultured as COC but not as DO.

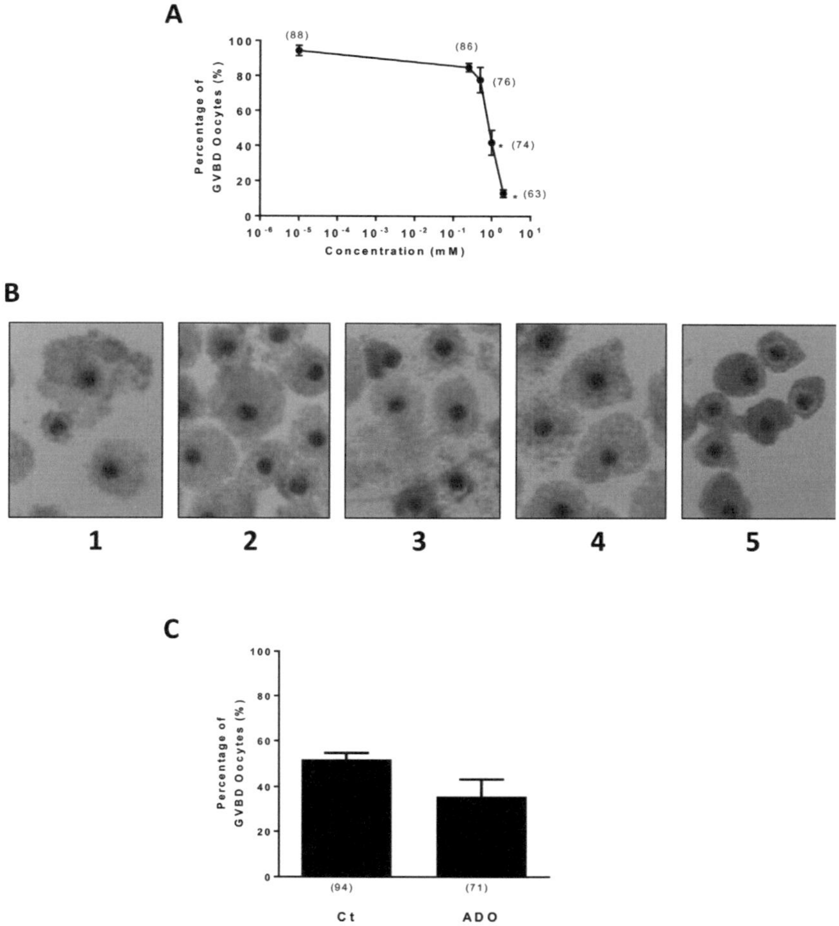

Figure 1.
*Dose-response of ADO on both (A) the percentage of GVBD oocyte and (B) cumulus cell expansion. (C) Effect of ADO (2.0 mM) on the percentage of denuded oocytes in GVBD. Data are presented as the mean ± SEM of a minimum of three replicates. The number of oocytes used is illustrated in parentheses. Statistically significant effect of the treatment at $P < 0.05$ is shown by *. In (B) treatments were (1) Ct, (2) ADO 0.25 mM, (3) ADO 0.5 mM, (4) ADO 1.0 mM, and (5) ADO 2.0 mM.*

3.2 Cell-permeable analog of adenosine (8-BrADO) inhibits GVBD

The following experiment is performed to assess a membrane-permeable analog of ADO, 8-BrADO (mimicking the intracellular effect). When COC are cultured for 24 hours, 12.2 ± 2.7% of the oocytes were in GVBD when treated with 2.0 mM ADO and 15.9 ± 0.8% when treated with 2.0 mM 8-BrADO (**Figure 2A**). These two treatments are significantly different to the control treatment (88.7 ± 2.9%; **Figure 2A**). The inhibition of cumulus cell expansion is also observed in both treatments (**Figure 2B2** and **B3**). These results support that the inhibitory effect of ADO may be mimicked by the cell-permeable analog of adenosine, 8-BrADO.

3.3 Reversibility of GVBD inhibition

To assess the reversibility, the test compounds (ADO and 8-BrADO) are washed out, and the COC are cultured under control conditions for a second 24-hour

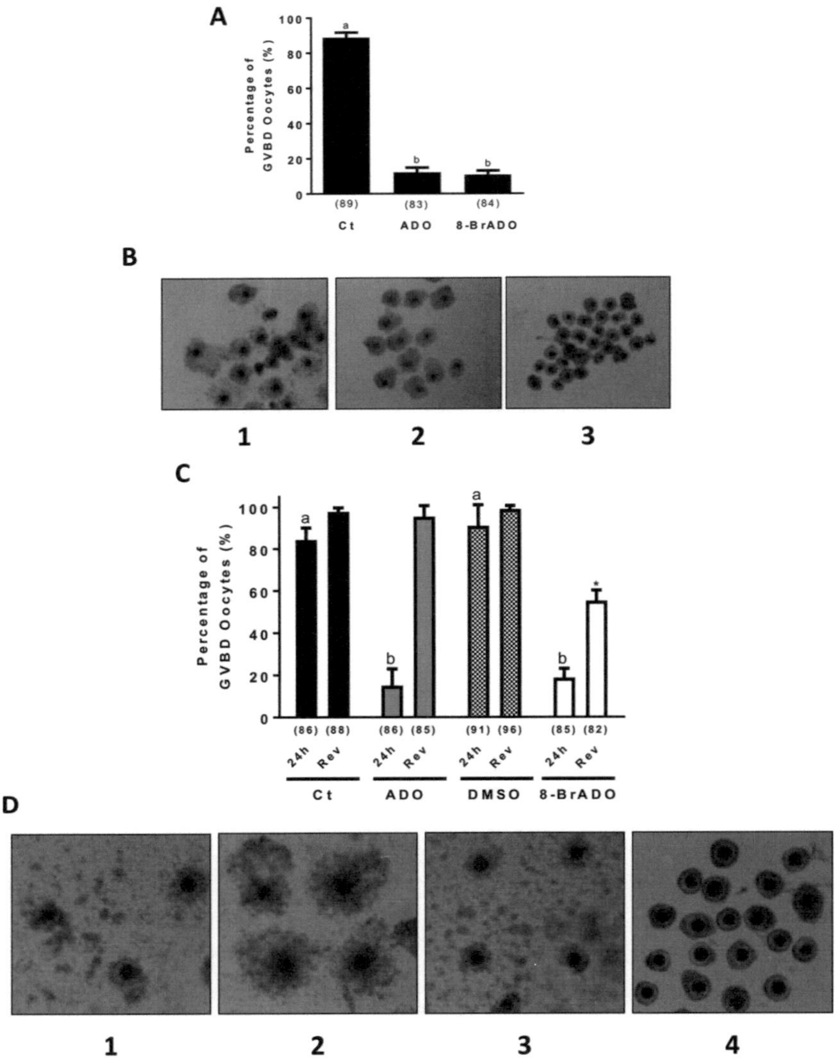

Figure 2.
*Comparison of the effect of ADO (2.0 mM) with the cell-permeable analog 8-BrADO (2.0 mM) on both the percentage of GVBD oocytes and cumulus cell expansion after (A–B) 24 hours and (C–D) reversibility of 24 hours (Rev). DMSO treatment at 0.1% is the control for 8-BrADO. (C) Reversibility: COC were first cultured for 24 hours according to treatment and then cultured for a second 24 hours in control culture medium (Ct) to assess the reversibility of the inhibition of oocyte meiotic resumption. Data are expressed as the mean ±SEM of a minimum of three replicates. The number of oocytes used is illustrated in parentheses. Statistically significant effect of treatment at P < 0.05 is shown by different letters and *. In (B), treatments were (1) Ct, (2) ADO, and (3) 8-BrADO. In (D) treatments were (1) Ct, (2) ADO, (3) DMSO, and (4) 8-BrADO.*

period. The ADO-treated oocytes resumed meiosis showing no statistical difference with the control treatment, whereas a significant lower percentage of GVBD oocytes is observed following treatment with 8-BrADO (**Figure 2C**). Cumulus cell expansion is compromised by 8-BrADO (**Figure 2D4**), supporting an impairment of oocyte maturation (nuclear maturation and cumulus cell expansion) when using the halogenate compound. However, cumulus cells are expanding following reversibility treatment of the ADO-treated COC (**Figure 2D2**), supporting the reversibility of the ADO inhibitory effect. The appropriate controls are presented in **Figure 2D1** and **D3**. These data are supportive of an adenosinergic system involved in the control of oocyte meiotic resumption.

3.4 Gap junction communications measured by cumulus-cumulus gap-FRAP assay

Since gap junction communications are highly regulated during in vitro maturation [17, 18], the aim of the following experiment was to measure the impact of

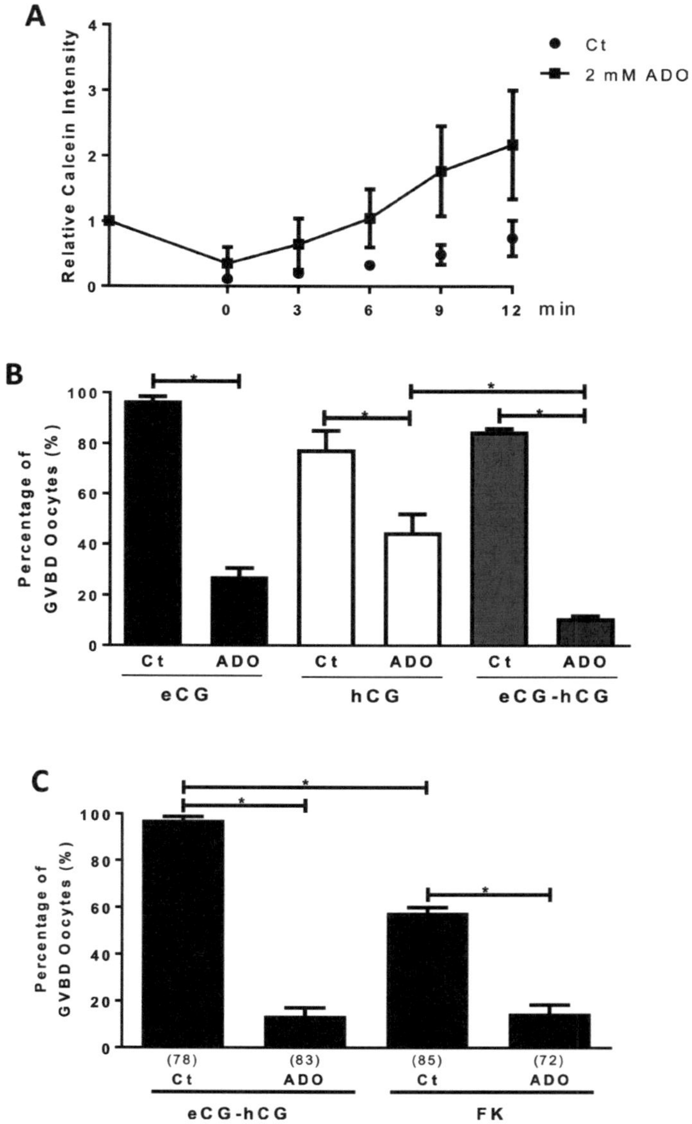

Figure 3.
*Effect of ADO (A) on gap junction communication, (B) according to hormonal supplementation, and (C) according to FK supplementation. (A) The effect of ADO (2.0 mM) on gap junction communications in between cumulus cells measured by fluorescent recovery after photobleaching after 4 hours of in vitro culture. The COC were prepared using calcein-AM as fluorescent probe. The data were plotted as relative intensity and presented as the mean ±SEM of a minimum of three replicates. ADO-treated cumulus cells recover significantly more fluorescence than the control cumulus cells (P < 0.05). (B) The effect of ADO according to hormonal supplementation on the percentage of GVBD oocyte after 24 hours of in vitro maturation. ADO (2.0 mM) was added either with eCG or hCG or both eCG and hCG. Data are expressed as the mean ± SEM of a minimum of three replicates. Statistically significant effect of the treatment at P < 0.05 is shown by *. (C) The effect of ADO (2.0 mM) in the presence of either eCG and hCG or the adenylyl cyclase activator forskolin (FK, 1.1 μM), for 24 hours on the percentage of GVBD oocyte. Data are expressed as the mean ± SEM of a minimum of three replicates. The number of oocytes used is illustrated in parentheses. Statistically significant effect of the treatment at P < 0.05 is shown by *.*

ADO treatment on gap junction communications measured by cumulus-cumulus gap-FRAP assay using calcein-AM as already described [12, 16]. Gap junction communication in cumulus cells was assessed after a 4-hour incubation in the presence of ADO (2.0 mM). The results show that gap junction communications between cumulus cells is increased following ADO treatment compared with the control treatment (**Figure 3A**). These results support that ADO maintains functional gap junctional communications between cumulus cells.

3.5 The contribution of eCG in adenosine treatment

The goal of the following experiment was to assess the contribution of gonadotropins in ADO-treated COC. The effect of ADO in inhibiting GVBD oocytes is observed in the presence of either eCG or hCG, or both in combination (**Figure 3B**). Comparison of ADO treatment supplemented with these hormones revealed no significant difference between eCG and the combination of eCG and hCG. However, a significant decrease in the percentage of GVBD was measured

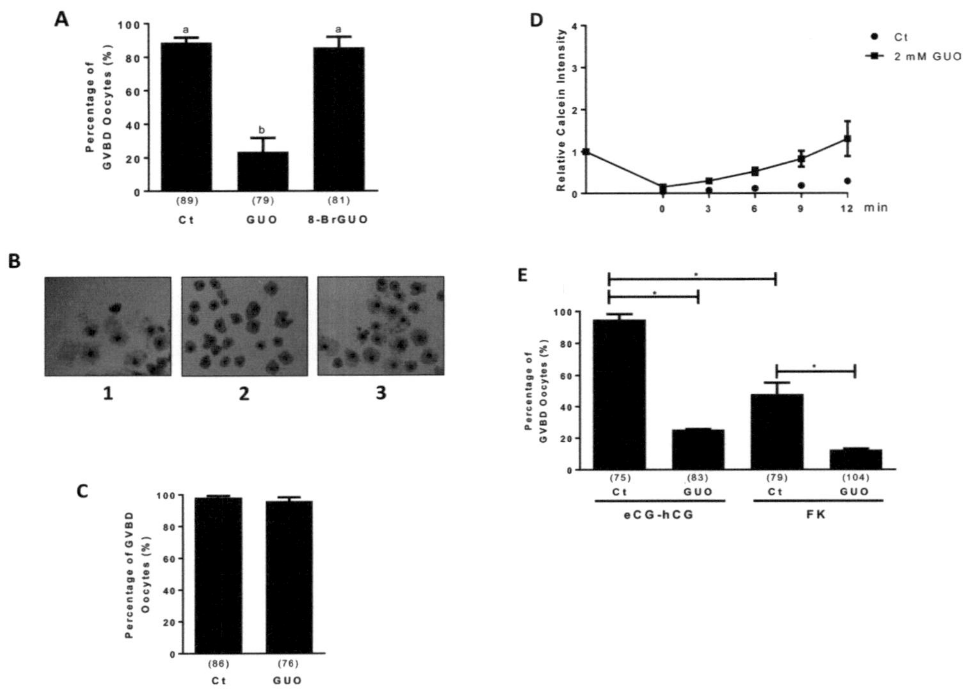

Figure 4.
*The effect of GUO (A) on the percentage of GVBD oocytes, (B) on cumulus cell expansion, (C) on reversibility, (D) on gap junction communication, and (E) according to FK supplementation. (A–B) Comparison of the effect of GUO (2.0 mM) and 8-BrGUO (2.0 mM) after 24 hours. (C) Reversibility: COC were first cultured for 24 hours in the presence of 2.0 mM of GUO and then cultured for a second 24 hours in control culture medium (Ct) to assess the reversibility of the inhibition of oocyte meiotic resumption. Data are expressed as the mean ± SEM of a minimum of three replicates. The number of oocytes used is illustrated in parentheses. Statistically significant effect of the treatment at P < 0.05 is shown by different letters. (D) The effect of GUO (2.0 mM) on gap junction communications in between cumulus cells measured by fluorescent recovery after photobleaching after 4 hours of in vitro culture. The data were plotted as relative intensity and presented as the mean ± SEM of a minimum of three replicates. GUO-treated cumulus cells recover significantly more fluorescence than the control cumulus cells (P < 0.05). (E) The effect of GUO (2.0 mM) in the presence of either eCG and hCG or the adenylyl cyclase activator forskolin (FK, 1.1 μM), for 24 hours on the percentage of GVBD oocyte. Data are expressed as the mean ± SEM of a minimum of three replicates. The number of oocytes used is illustrated in parentheses. Statistically significant effect of the treatment at P < 0.05 is shown by *. In (B), treatments were (1) Ct, (2) GUO, and (3) 8-BrGUO.*

between hCG alone and the combination of hCG and eCG (**Figure 3B**), showing the significant contribution of eCG to ADO-inhibiting GVBD, yet supporting an adenosinergic system.

3.6 Adenylyl cyclase activator (forskolin)

Since eCG contributes to ADO inhibitory effect, the following experiment was to evaluate the involvement of cAMP while using the adenylyl cyclase activator, forskolin. On itself, forskolin is significantly decreasing the percentage of GVBD oocytes (**Figure 3C**). ADO was significantly inhibiting GVBD both in presence of eCG-hCG and forskolin (**Figure 3C**). However, forskolin was not significantly

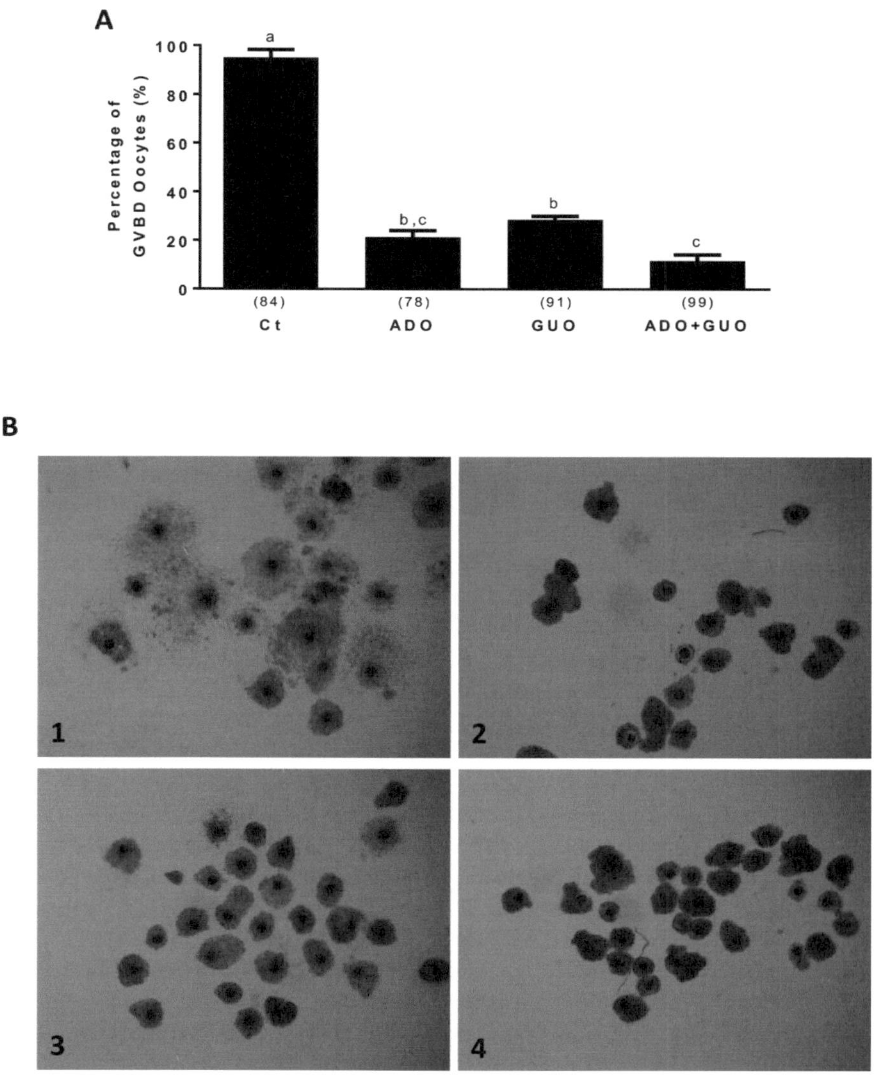

Figure 5.
The effect of supplementing both ADO and GUO (2.0 mM each) on (A) the percentage of oocyte meiotic resumption and (B) cumulus cell expansion. Data are expressed as the mean ± SEM of a minimum of three replicates. The number of oocytes used is illustrated in parentheses. Statistically significant effect of the treatment at P < 0.05 is shown by different letters. (B) The treatments were (1) Ct, (2) ADO 2.0 mM, (3) GUO 2.0 mM, (4) ADO 2.0 mM and GUO 2.0 mM.

changing the percentage of GVBD compared with eCG-hCG (**Figure 3C**). The results are proposing the contribution of cAMP to ADO-inhibiting GVBD.

3.7 Guanosine inhibits oocyte meiotic resumption

High-performance liquid chromatography was used to detect the presence of GUO in porcine follicular fluid from follicles of 2–6 mm in diameter (data not shown). Since GUO was detected in PFF, we undertook to assess whether GUO could play a role in inhibiting GVBD. **Figure 4** shows the significant effect of GUO in inhibiting both GVBD and cumulus expansion after 24 hours, highlighting the contribution of GUO in oocyte maturation. However, the membrane-permeable analog 8-BrGUO did not significantly inhibit GVBD (**Figure 4A**). Cumulus cell expansion was observed (**Figure 4B3**), supporting the inefficacy of 8-BrGUO in inhibiting oocyte GVBD and cumulus cell expansion. The reversibility treatment showed that GUO-treated COC resumed meiosis without any statistical significance compared with the control treatment (**Figure 4C**), supporting the reversibility of GUO inhibitory effect on GVBD. As ADO, GUO was also significantly increasing gap junction communication as measured by gap-FRAP assay (**Figure 4D**). Finally, forskolin was not significantly improving the inhibitory effect of GUO compared to eCG-hCG supplementation as measured on the percentage of GVBD oocytes (**Figure 4E**). GUO was also reversibly inhibiting oocyte GVBD, thus supporting a guanosinergic system.

3.8 The effect of using both ADO and GUO

The final experiment evaluated the effect of supplementing both ADO and GUO at 2.0 mM each on GVBD oocytes using COC (**Figure 5A**). The results showed that ADO, GUO, and both ADO and GUO were all significantly decreasing GVDB percentage compared with the control treatment. Although a significant effect of adding ADO with GUO was observed when compared with GUO (**Figure 5A**), the impact on the percentage went from 28.6 ± 1.4% for GUO to 11.8 ± 2.5% for ADO and GUO. Cumulus cell expansion was inhibited by ADO (**Figure 5B2**), GUO (**Figure 5B3**), and the combination of ADO and GUO (**Figure 5B4**) when compared with the control (**Figure 5B1**).

4. Discussion

The present study showed that both ADO and GUO are efficient in reversibly inhibiting swine oocyte GVBD (**Figures 1** and **4**). Cumulus cell expansion is significantly inhibited after 24 hours in presence to either ADO or GUO (**Figures 1** and **4**), supporting that these two purine nucleosides inhibit oocyte maturation with low GVBD percentages and no cumulus cell expansion. Both ADO and GUO also increased GJC in cumulus cells (**Figures 3** and **4**). eCG and FK are both supporting the two purines' inhibitory effect (**Figures 3** and **4**). The data suggest that the inhibitory effect of these two purines on GVBD strengthens the involvement of both adenosinergic and guanosinergic systems in meiotic resumption.

Several years ago it was clearly shown that hypoxanthine, a purine derivative, was an important component of a low molecular weight fraction from porcine follicular fluid and efficient at inhibiting oocyte GVBD [19]. It was also reported that this fraction did not exclusively contain hypoxanthine [10]. Although hypoxanthine was efficient in the mouse and rat, the question was still not fully assessed regarding the efficacy of ADO and GUO on swine COC with respect to the inhibition of oocyte meiotic resumption.

From a broader perspective, it is known that ADO is involved in several biological functions such as nucleotide biosynthesis and cellular energy metabolism [19]. The cellular uptake of ADO played by two classes of nucleotide transporters (SLC28 and SLC29) regulates these biological functions. Inside the cell, ADO is rapidly metabolized and either converted to inosine or adenosine monophosphate through adenosine deaminase or adenosine kinase, respectively [20]. Alternatively, extracellular ADO may serve as a signaling molecule, which activates adenosine receptors (ADORA) on the cell membrane surface. Four different seven-transmembrane domain receptors have been described [21]. It has been reported that a low dose of ADO (0.2 mM) produced a transient delay in bovine oocyte GVBD [9]. After 21 hours in culture, neither ADO nor hypoxanthine resulted in an efficient inhibition of oocyte GVBD [9]. In the mouse, 4.0 mM of hypoxanthine was clearly efficient at inhibiting oocyte GVBD, while the use of ADO by itself did not produce a significant inhibition [10]. However, the efficacy was enhanced when ADO was used in combination with hypoxanthine [7]. This was also observed when ADO was used together with FSH [22], forskolin [23], or cAMP analogs such as 8-bromo-cAMP [8]. Although these results have been provided to support that adenosine uptake and metabolism contribute to the inhibition of GVBD [24], ample evidence shows that functional adenosine receptors are present on ovarian cells [25]. The measured concentration of ADO in murine follicular fluid was between 0.38 and 0.68 mM [7]. In the present study, the inhibitory effect on GVBD was dose-dependent with an IC_{50} of 1.3 mM (**Figure 1**). Using 2.0 mM, ADO was efficient at reversibly inhibiting swine oocyte GVBD and cumulus cell expansion (**Figure 1**).

Although hypoxanthine and ADO have been measured in PFF [10], GUO has never been reported. In the present study, GUO has been found in PFF from 2 to 6 mm diameter follicles (data not shown). While limited information is available in the literature regarding GUO, it has been described as having important functions as an intercellular messenger especially in the central nervous system [4]. The mechanism underlying the neuroprotective properties of GUO is still not fully understood. One working hypothesis is that GUO may exert its biological effect by synchronizing distinct signaling pathways that may be related to the activation of purinergic receptor and specific G-protein binding sites [26–28]. In this study, 2.0 mM of GUO is reversibly inhibiting GVBD and cumulus cell expansion (**Figure 5**). In the mouse, GUO (1.0 mM) was reported to inhibit GVBD, while the same concentration of either hypoxanthine or ADO was inefficient [10]. In rats, the reported order of potency of these nucleosides was GUO > hypoxanthine > ADO [8]. In the mouse, there is an assumption based on a synergistic effect of ADO and GUO on the inhibition oocyte GVBD [7]. In the present study, the combination at 2.0 mM significantly increased the effect of GUO (**Figure 5**). Thus, the inhibitory effect of the combination of both ADO and GUO are somewhat additive according to the concentration used. Although GUO is proposed to activate a specific G-protein-coupled receptor with the involvement of P1 receptor [29], it has been recently reported that GUO functions as an extracellular signaling molecule without the need for GUO receptors [30]. In vascular smooth muscle cells, extracellular GUO regulated extracellular ADO [30]. This proposed GUO-ADO mechanism further regulated cell proliferation in vitro [31] and decreased inflammation in vivo [32], supporting the additive inhibitory effect observed on oocyte GVBD.

We recently demonstrated the regulation of gap junction communications between cumulus cells during in vitro maturation [16–18]. An increase in gap junction communication was evident after 4 hours of in vitro culture [17, 18]. This observation provides an indication of how cumulus cells respond to the treatment and not only looking at cumulus cell expansion. In the present study, the effect of both treatments, ADO and GUO, was to increase gap junction communications compared with the control (**Figures 3** and **4**). Since gap junction communications are known to play a primordial role in oocyte maturation [33, 34], this result supports a clear impact of the treatments on cumulus cell functions that may be beneficial for the oocyte.

This study also provides evidence of hormonal supplementation impacting the inhibition of GVBD oocytes by ADO (**Figure 3**). This ADO-mediated inhibition of GVBD oocytes is improved according to the supplementation. Although it is not the purpose of this study to understand how this effect is transduced into the cells, eCG clearly improved the effect of ADO in the presence of hCG. This FSH-type stimulation seemed to be sufficient since the effect of eCG alone was not significantly different from that of eCG and hCG (**Figure 3**). As it is well-known that cumulus cells have an efficient response to FSH [35, 36], the inhibitory effect of ADO is significantly increased by FSH. This effect has been reported in the rat where the percentage of GVBD oocyte treated with ADO was decreased in the presence of FSH [22]. In addition, the FSH-induced granulosa cell differentiation was reduced by ADO [37], supporting the involvement of ADO in FSH response.

Although different forms of adenylyl cyclase have been characterized in oocytes and in cumulus cells [38], forskolin, a known adenylyl cyclase activator, makes a significant contribution to the inhibition of spontaneous maturation in several species as observed for rat [39], bovine [40], and porcine [11] oocytes. In the present study, forskolin inhibited oocyte GVBD while treated with ADO (**Figure 3C**). Similar results were obtained in the presence of GUO (**Figure 4E**). These results support that constant stimulation of adenylyl cyclase, which increases the intracellular concentration of cAMP [40], promoted the inhibitory effects of ADO and GUO. In this regard, the results are proposing the contribution of cAMP to both ADO- and GUO-inhibiting GVBD.

The effect of the two purines goes well with the current working model of inhibition of oocyte GVBD involving C-type natriuretic peptide (CNP) as an oocyte-meiosis-inhibiting peptide [41, 42]. CNP is involved in inhibiting oocyte GVBD [41, 43, 44]. CNP produced by granulosa cells is a ligand for NPR2, a member of guanylyl cyclase receptor family. NPR2 stimulation by CNP increased intracellular concentration of cGMP, inhibited oocyte phosphodiesterase type 3A, and thus maintained high intra-oocyte concentration of cAMP. The contribution of both purine nucleosides supports adenosinergic and guanosinergic system in the inhibition of oocyte meiotic resumption.

5. Conclusion

In conclusion, this study puts forward the contribution of ADO and GUO as inhibitory for oocyte GVBD in vitro suggesting that both adenosinergic and guanosinergic systems are efficient in inhibiting oocyte meiotic resumption. The use of these two systems as part of a pre-IVM culture period would be a novel strategy to explore in order to improve oocyte developmental competence.

Finally, it should be emphasized that the signaling involved in oocyte meiotic resumption may be modulated through the contribution of different pathways. The adenosinergic and guanosinergic systems of which we have presented the contribution illustrate this situation for meiotic resumption. It is also to be expected that other studies will pave the way for additional contributions. For example, a preliminary study from our lab revealed that, as demonstrated in bovine [45], porcine theca cells secreted efficient factors involved in oocyte meiotic resumption. Without knowing these secreted elements, this result highlights that oocyte meiotic resumption is under the control of the ovarian follicular cells. Meiotic resumption is thus under high surveillance!

Acknowledgements

This work was supported by the Natural Sciences and Engineering Research Council of Canada (RGPIN-2014-04774). Appreciation is extended to Mario Mayes for his contribution to the experimental work.

Conflict of interest

The author has no conflict of interest to declare.

Author details

François J. Richard
Centre de recherche en reproduction, développement et santé intergénérationnelle, Département des Sciences Animales, Faculté des sciences de l'agriculture et de l'alimentation, Université Laval, Québec, Québec, Canada

*Address all correspondence to: francois.richard@fsaa.ulaval.ca

References

[1] Colledge WH, Carlton MBL, Udy GB, Evans MJ. Disruption of c-mos causes parthenogenetic development of unfertilized mouse eggs. Nature. 1994;**370**:65. DOI: 10.1038/370065a0

[2] Benarroch EE. Adenosine and its receptors: Multiple modulatory functions and potential therapeutic targets for neurologic disease. Neurology. 2008;**70**:231-236. DOI: 10.1212/01.wnl.0000297939.18236.ec

[3] Haskó G. Adenosine: An endogenous regulator of innate immunity. Trends in Immunology. 2004;**25**:33-39. DOI: 10.1016/j.it.2003.11.003

[4] Lanznaster D, Dal-Cim T, Piermartiri TC, Tasca CI. Guanosine: A neuromodulator with therapeutic potential in brain disorders. Aging and Disease. 2016;**7**:657-679. DOI: 10.14336/AD.2016.0208

[5] Lanznaster D, Tasca CI. Targeting the guanine-based purinergic system in Alzheimer's disease. Neural Regeneration Research. 2017;**12**:212-213. DOI: 10.4103/1673-5374.200801

[6] Dubyak GR, el-Moatassim C. Signal transduction via P2-purinergic receptors for extracellular ATP and other nucleotides. The American Journal of Physiology. 1993;**265**:C577-C606. DOI: 10.1152/ajpcell.1993.265.3.C577

[7] Eppig JJ, Ward-Bailey PF, Coleman DL. Hypoxanthine and adenosine in murine ovarian follicular fluid: Concentrations and activity in maintaining oocyte meiotic arrest. Biology of Reproduction. 1985;**33**:1041-1049. DOI: 10.1095/biolreprod33.5.1041

[8] Tornell J, Brannstrom M, Magnusson C, Billig H. Effects of follicle stimulating hormone and purines on rat oocyte maturation. Molecular Reproduction and Development. 1990;**27**:254-260. DOI: 10.1002/mrd.1080270312

[9] Sirard MA, First NL. In vitro inhibition of oocyte nuclear maturation in the bovine. Biology of Reproduction. 1988;**39**:229-234. DOI: 10.1095/biolreprod39.2.229

[10] Downs SM, Coleman DL, Ward-Bailey PF, Eppig JJ. Hypoxanthine is the principal inhibitor of murine oocyte maturation in a low molecular weight fraction of porcine follicular fluid. Proceedings of the National Academy of Sciences of the United States of America. 1985;**82**:454-458. DOI: 10.1073/pnas.82.2.454

[11] Laforest MF, Pouliot É, Guéguen L, Richard FJ. Fundamental significance of specific phosphodiesterases in the control of spontaneous meiotic resumption in porcine oocytes. Molecular Reproduction and Development. 2005;**70**:361-372. DOI: 10.1002/mrd.20203

[12] Santiquet N, Sasseville M, Laforest M, Guillemette C, Gilchrist RB, Richard FJ. Activation of 5′ adenosine monophosphate-activated protein kinase blocks cumulus cell expansion through inhibition of protein synthesis during in vitro maturation in swine. Biology of Reproduction. 2014;**91**:51. DOI: 10.1095/biolreprod.113.116764

[13] Petters RM, Wells KD. Culture of pig embryos. Journal of Reproduction and Fertility. Supplement. 1993;**48**:61-73

[14] Funahashi H, Koike T, Sakai R. Effect of glucose and pyruvate on nuclear and cytoplasmic maturation of porcine oocytes in a chemically defined medium. Theriogenology. 2008;**70**:1041-1047. DOI: 10.1016/j.theriogenology.2008.06.025

[15] Motlík J, Fulka J. Breakdown of the germinal vesicle in pig oocytes

in vivo and in vitro. The Journal of Experimental Zoology. 1976;**198**:155-162. DOI: 10.1002/jez.1401980205

[16] Sasseville M, Gagnon M-C, Guillemette C, Sullivan R, Gilchrist RB, Richard FJ. Regulation of gap junctions in porcine cumulus-oocyte complexes: Contributions of granulosa cell contact, gonadotropins, and lipid rafts. Molecular Endocrinology. 2009;**23**:700-710. DOI: 10.1210/me.2008-0320

[17] Santiquet NW, Develle Y, Laroche A, Robert C, Richard FJ. Regulation of gap-junctional communication between cumulus cells during in vitro maturation in swine, a gap-FRAP study. Biology of Reproduction. 2012;**87**:46. DOI: 10.1095/biolreprod.112.099754

[18] Santiquet N, Robert C, Richard FJ. The dynamics of connexin expression, degradation and localisation are regulated by gonadotropins during the early stages of in vitro maturation of swine oocytes. PLoS ONE. 2013;**8**:e68456. DOI: 10.1371/journal.pone.0068456

[19] Young JD, Yao SY, Baldwin JM, Cass CE, Baldwin SA. The human concentrative and equilibrative nucleoside transporter families, SLC28 and SLC29. Molecular Aspects of Medicine. 2013;**34**:529-547. DOI: 10.1016/j.mam.2012.05.007

[20] Eltzschig HK. Adenosine: An old drug newly discovered. Anesthesiology. 2009;**111**:904-915. DOI: 10.1097/ALN.0b013e3181b060f2

[21] Linden J. Molecular approach to adenosine receptors: Receptor-mediated mechanisms of tissue protection. Annual Review of Pharmacology and Toxicology. 2001;**41**:775-787. DOI: 10.1146/annurev.pharmtox.41.1.775

[22] Miller JG, Behrman HR. Oocyte maturation is inhibited by adenosine in the presence of follicle-stimulating hormone. Biology of Reproduction. 1986;**35**:833-837. DOI: 10.1095/biolreprod35.4.833

[23] Salustri A, Petrungaro S, Conti M, Siracusa G. Adenosine potentiates forskolin-induced delay of meiotic resumption by mouse denuded oocytes: Evidence for an oocyte surface site of adenosine action. Gamete Research. 1988;**21**:157-168. DOI: 10.1002/mrd.1120210206

[24] Downs SM. Uptake and metabolism of adenosine mediate a meiosis-arresting action on mouse oocytes. Molecular Reproduction and Development. 1999;**53**:208-221. DOI: 10.1002/(SICI)1098-2795(199906)53:2<208::AID-MRD10>3.0.CO;2-O

[25] Billig H, Rosberg S, Johanson C, Ahren K. Adenosine as substrate and receptor agonist in the ovary. Steroids. 1989;**54**:523-542

[26] Ciccarelli R, Ballerini P, Sabatino G, Rathbone MP, D'Onofrio M, Caciagli F, et al. Involvement of astrocytes in purine-mediated reparative processes in the brain. International Journal of Developmental Neuroscience. 2001;**19**:395-414. DOI: 10.1016/S0736-5748(00)00084-8

[27] Thauerer B, Zur Nedden S, Baier-Bitterlich G. Purine nucleosides: Endogenous neuroprotectants in hypoxic brain. Journal of Neurochemistry. 2012;**121**:329-342. DOI: 10.1111/j.1471-4159.2012.07692.x

[28] Ciruela F. Guanosine behind the scene. Journal of Neurochemistry. 2013;**126**:425-427. DOI: 10.1111/jnc.12328

[29] Bettio LEB, Gil-Mohapel J, Rodrigues ALS. Guanosine and its role in neuropathologies. Purinergic Signal. 2016;**12**:411-426. DOI: 10.1007/s11302-016-9509-4

[30] Jackson EK, Cheng D, Jackson TC, Verrier JD, Gillespie DG. Extracellular guanosine regulates extracellular adenosine levels. American Journal of Physiology. Cell Physiology. 2013;**304**:C406-C421. DOI: 10.1152/ajpcell.00212.2012

[31] Jackson EK, Gillespie DG. Regulation of cell proliferation by the guanosine-adenosine mechanism: Role of adenosine receptors. Physiological Reports. 2013;**1**:e00024. DOI: 10.1002/phy2.24

[32] Jackson EK, Mi Z. The guanosine-adenosine interaction exists in vivo. The Journal of Pharmacology and Experimental Therapeutics. 2014;**350**: 719-726. DOI: 10.1124/jpet.114.216978

[33] Gershon E, Plaks V, Aharon I, Galiani D, Reizel Y, Sela-Abramovich S, et al. Oocyte-directed depletion of connexin43 using the Cre-LoxP system leads to subfertility in female mice. Developmental Biology. 2008;**313**:1-12. DOI: 10.1016/j.ydbio.2007.08.041

[34] Conti M, Hsieh M, Musa Zamah A, Oh JS. Novel signaling mechanisms in the ovary during oocyte maturation and ovulation. Molecular and Cellular Endocrinology. 2012;**356**:65-73. DOI: 10.1016/j.mce.2011.11.002

[35] Khan DR, Guillemette C, Sirard MA, Richard FJ. Characterization of FSH signalling networks in bovine cumulus cells: A perspective on oocyte competence acquisition. Molecular Human Reproduction. 2015;**21**:688-701. DOI: 10.1093/molehr/gav032

[36] Ali A, Sirard MA. Protein kinases influence bovine oocyte competence during short-term treatment with recombinant human follicle stimulating hormone. Reproduction. 2005;**130**:303-310. DOI: 10.1530/rep.1.00387

[37] Knecht M, Darbon JM, Ranta T, Baukal A, Catt KJ. Inhibitory actions of adenosine on follicle-stimulating hormone-induced differentiation of cultured rat granulosa cells. Biology of Reproduction. 1984;**30**:1082-1090. DOI: 10.1095/biolreprod30.5.1082

[38] Horner K, Livera G, Hinckley M, Trinh K, Storm D, Conti M. Rodent oocytes express an active adenylyl cyclase required for meiotic arrest. Developmental Biology. 2003;**258**:385-396. DOI: 10.1016/s0012-1606(03)00134-9

[39] Dekel N, Aberdam E, Sherizly I. Spontaneous maturation in vitro of cumulus-enclosed rat oocytes is inhibited by forskolin. Biology of Reproduction. 1984;**31**:244-250. DOI: 10.1095/biolreprod31.2.244

[40] Bilodeau S, Fortier MA, Sirard MA. Effect of adenylate cyclase stimulation on meiotic resumption and cyclic AMP content of zona-free and cumulus-enclosed bovine oocytes in vitro. Reproduction. 1993;**97**:5-11. DOI: 10.1530/jrf.0.0970005

[41] Zhang M, Su YQ, Sugiura K, Xia G, Eppig JJ. Granulosa cell ligand NPPC and its receptor NPR2 maintain meiotic arrest in mouse oocytes. Science. 2010;**330**:366-369. DOI: 10.1126/science.1193573

[42] Gilchrist RB, Luciano AM, Richani D, Zeng HT, Wang X, De Vos M, et al. Oocyte maturation and quality: Role of cyclic nucleotides. Reproduction. 2016;**152**:R143-R157. DOI: 10.1530/REP-15-0606

[43] Santiquet N, Papillon-Dion É, Djender N, Guillemette C, Richard FJ. New elements in the c-type natriuretic peptide signaling pathway inhibiting swine in vitro oocyte meiotic resumption. Biology of Reproduction. 2014;**91**:16. DOI: 10.1095/biolreprod.113.114132

[44] Franciosi F, Coticchio G, Lodde V, Tessaro I, Modina SC, Fadini R, et al.

Natriuretic peptide precursor C delays meiotic resumption and sustains gap junction-mediated communication in bovine cumulus-enclosed oocytes. Biology of Reproduction. 2014;**91**:61. DOI: 10.1095/biolreprod.114.118869

[45] Richard FJ, Sirard MA. Effects of follicular cells on oocyte maturation. II: Theca cell inhibition of bovine oocyte maturation in vitro. Biology of Reproduction. 1996;**54**:22-28. DOI: 10.1095/biolreprod54.1.22

Chapter 3

Effect of Pre and Post Weaning Diet Quality on Puberty Age and Tail Measures in Kurdish Female Lambs

Sedigheh Menatian, Hamidreza Mirzaei Alamouti, Farshid Fatahnia and Reza Masoumi

Abstract

To determine the value of pre and post weaning nutrition on puberty age, some hormonal concentrations and tail measures in ewe lambs, a total of 40 clinically health Kurdish female lambs (30±8.6 d and weighing 10.2±3.4 kg) were randomly allocated to one of two experimental diets in pre-weaning period: high quality diet (**HQD**, 2.50 Mcal ME/kg dry matter (**DM**) and 148 g CP/kg DM) or low quality diet (LQD, 2.02 Mcal ME/kg DM and 87 g CP/kg DM). At weaning, one half of lambs from each group was randomly separated and assigned to HQD or LQD. So there were four treatment groups in post-weaning period: H-H (HQD pre- and post-weaning); H-L (HQD pre-weaning and LQD post-weaning); L-H (LQD pre-weaning and HQD post-weaning) and L-L (LQD pre and post-weaning, control group). Within the post-weaning, serum progesterone concentrations was greater for ewe lambs fed at H-H group than for other groups ($P<0.05$). Serum insulin concentration was affected by the diet quality at both periods ($P<0.05$). Leptin concentration was affected by treatment and ewe lambs of L-H group had higher leptin concentrations ($P<0.05$). Diet plan in the pre-pubertal period was affected tail measures in 120 and 210 days of ages ($P<0.05$).

Keywords: hormone, Kurdish lambs, milk, nutrition plan, reproductive performance

1. Introduction

In tropical, semiarid, and arid areas, animal production is dependent on supplemental feeding, especially in the reproductive seasons due to the higher energy demand [1]. Reproduction efficiency can play a critical role in determining profit potential for livestock production systems. Most sheep breeds become sexually active in response to decreasing day length in the late summer to early autumn, which is an additional constraint to the timing of puberty in ewe lambs [2]. If a ewe lamb fails to achieve puberty in its first autumn, it will be delayed until the following breeding [3]. Breeding ewes to lamb at 1 year of age is a potential means of improving farm profitability and ewe lifetime performance by reducing the time interval from birth to first lambing, subsequently reducing feed, labor, housing, and other costs associated with raising replacement animals [4, 5].

Sexual development is an important factor and can be manipulated by altering growth rates [6–8]. During the productive life of ewes, puberty period is critical for both animal health and performance. The onset of puberty in sheep is influenced by genetic and environmental factors such as nutrition, day length, temperature, and their interaction [9]. Ewe lambs growing at faster rates will exhibit their first estrus and are more likely to conceive at a lower age and have heavier body weight (BW) than ewe lambs growing at slower rates [10]. Because of the importance of BW, environmental factors that can affect the rate of growth before and after weaning are important determinants of age at puberty. Mulvaney et al. [11] reported that ewe lambs gaining 208 g/day compared to 153 g/day were more likely to return to breeding, although overall pregnancy rates did not differ. Generally, faster growth is associated with enhanced reproductive performance in ewe lambs, i.e., earlier attainment of puberty, more intense estrous activity, and higher conception and lambing rates when mated [12].

The most economically important traits in sheep production are growth, reproductive performance, and milk production, and there is no study on the abovementioned characteristics in Kurdish ewe lambs; therefore, the objective of this study was to compare the effects of diet quality fed during the pre-weaning and post-weaning periods and potential interactions between pre- and post-weaning diets on skeletal growth, reproduction performance, hormone concentrations, and milk production during the first lactation in Kurdish ewe lambs.

2. Materials and methods

2.1 Hormonal drugs

Controlled internal drug release (CIDR) with 300 mg of progesterone, a progestagen analogue (InterAg, Hamilton, New Zealand), PMSG (Folligon; Intervet International BV, Boxmeer, the Netherlands), oxytocin (Oxytocin V, 10 IU/ml, Phoenix Pharm, Auckland, New Zealand), and commercially available kits of leptin (LDN, Germany, LOT: 150873), insulin (DiaMetra, Italy, LOT N: 3949C), and progesterone (DiaMetra. Italy. LOT N: 4026) were used.

2.2 Locations, animals, and treatment schedule

This study was performed at the Nomadic Management Department, Ilam Province, Iran (33°51′ N, 46°27′ E), from January 2013 to December 2015. All procedures involving animal care and management were approved by the University of Zanjan Animal Care Committee (proposal no. 1169739). A total of 40 clinically health Kurdish female lambs (30 ± 8.6 days and weighing 10.2 ± 3.4 kg) were used. At 30 days of age, lambs were randomly housed together with twice daily access to their mother's milk and were allocated to one of the two experimental treatments to achieve either high or low rates of BW gain during two consecutive periods, from 30 to 120 (pre-weaning period) and from 121 to 210 days of age (post-weaning period). They were kept in individual pens (1 × 2 m) for three consecutive days every 2 weeks for recording dry matter intake (DMI). In pre-weaning period, the lambs were fed high-quality diet (HQD, n = 20) or low-quality diet (LQD, n = 20), and at the weaning time, HQD and LQD fed lambs were re-randomized so that one half of lambs from each group is randomly allocated to HQD or LQD. So there were four treatment groups (n = 10) in post-weaning period: HQD pre- and post-weaning (H-H); HQD pre-weaning and LQD post-weaning (H-L); LQD pre-weaning and

Composition (%)	Pre- and post-weaning diets	
	HQD	LQD
Alfalfa hay	445.1	—
Wheat straw	—	513.7
Ground barley	445.1	428.1
Soybean meal	59.3	—
Calcium carbonate	5.9	6.8
Salt	5.0	5.0
Mineral and vitamin premix*	39.6	46.4
DM	916.0	919.0
CP	148.0	87.0
EE	58.0	22.0
NDF	285.0	450.0
NFC	466.0	371.0
ME (Mcal/kg)	2.50	2.02

Pre- and post-weaning treatments: HQD, high-quality diet; LQD, low-quality diet.
**Each kg (DM basis) of mineral and vitamin premix contained 180 g of Ca, 70 g of P, 35 g of K, 50 g of Na, 58 g of Cl, 30 g of Mg, 32 g of S, 5 g of Mn, 4 g of Fe, 3 g of Zn, 300 mg of Cu, 100 mg of I, 100 mg of Co, 20 mg of Se, 400,000 IU vitamin A, 100,000 IU vitamin D3, and 245 IU vitamin E. DM, dry matter; CP, crude protein; EE, ether extract; NFC, nonfiber carbohydrates = 100 − (CP + NDF + EE + ash); ME, metabolite energy.*

Table 1.
Ingredients and chemical composition of experimental diets.

HQD post-weaning (L-H); and LQD pre- and post-weaning (L-L, control group). The HQD and LQD were formulated according to recommended nutrient requirements for small ruminants [13] that received a diet that covered nutrient requirements including energy and protein needs for a 20 kg growing lamb with an average daily gain (ADG) of 200 and 100 g/day, respectively. Diets were formulated to have different metabolize energy (ME) and crude protein (CP) contents. The HQD and LQD were contained 2.50 and 2.02 Mcal ME /kg DM and 14.9 and 8.9% CP (DM basis), respectively. Rations were totally hand-mixed for each pen and offered in equal proportions twice daily at 09:00 and 16:00 in pre- and post-weaning period. The ingredients and chemical composition of the experimental diets are shown in **Table 1.**

2.3 Estrous synchronization and pregnancy diagnosis

When ewe lambs reached 210 days old, estrus was induced and synchronized by CIDR. Animals were treated with CIDR for 14 days and were injected with 500 IU PMSG at the time of CIDR withdrawal. Twenty-four hours after CIDR withdrawal, all of ewe lambs were monitored for estrus detection by five intact fertile rams and were ultimately naturally bred. The rams remained with the ewe lambs until the termination of estrous signs. After serving, all ewe lambs were kept together in the same nutritional and managerial conditions and reared in the pasture until 2 weeks before expected parturition. Pregnancy diagnosis was determined by using of transabdominal ultrasound (Pie Medical, Falco 100, Netherlands) at 60 days after serving.

2.4 Data collection and calculation

BW was measured every 2 weeks from 30 to 210 days of age. Feed offered and feed refusals of individual pens were weighed and recorded daily, and DM content of total mixed ration (TMR) and orts was determined to estimate DMI. ME and CP intake were calculated as DMI from each diet multiplied by their ME and CP contents, respectively [13]. DM, CP, and ether extract (EE) of experimental diets were measured according to the methods of AOAC [14]. The neutral detergent fiber (NDF) was measured according to the method described by Van Soest et al. [15] without α-amylase and sodium sulfite and was expressed exclusive of residual ash. Nonfibrous carbohydrates (NFC) were calculated according to NRC [16] dairy cattle model as 100 − (CP + NDF + EE + ash). Milk intake by ewe lambs was measured by the weigh-suckle-weigh method (WSW) in three consecutive days every 2 weeks from the start of study to weaning (30–120 days). At the start of WSW method at each suckling occasion (twice daily), ewe lambs were weighed, allowed to suckle the udder of their dams, and weighed again immediately after suckling. The difference between pre- and post-suckling weights was defined as milk intake (2 months [17]). On each milking occasion, ewes were milked by hand after intravenous injection of 1 IU synthetic oxytocin. Milk samples of dams in subsequent lactation were collected in three consecutive days every 2 weeks and analyzed for fat, protein, and lactose by using of MilkoScan 133B (Foss Electric, Hillerød, Denmark). Milk protein, fat, and lactose yields were calculated by multiplying milk yield from the respective day by protein, fat, and lactose contents of the milk for each ewe. Milk gross energy (GE) was calculated as GE = ((0.0547 × CP%) + (0.0929 × Fat%) + (0.0395 × Lactose%)) according to NRC [16]. The mean metabolize ability of the ewe milk GE is 0.94 [18]; therefore, milk ME content was calculated as GE × 0.94. Energy-corrected milk (ECM) and fat-corrected milk (6.5% FCM) were calculated as ECM = (0.327 × kg milk) + (12.95 × kg fat) + (7.2 × kg protein) and FCM = milk yield × (0.37 + (0.097 × Fat%)).

2.5 Blood sampling and analysis

Before the first meal of the day, blood samples (5 ml) were collected by jugular venipuncture from each lamb every 2 weeks from 90 days of age until puberty (age at puberty was assessed by serum concentrations of progesterone, where puberty was determined as the age when two consecutive blood samples contained at least 1 ng of progesterone/mL). Hence, samples were centrifuged for 15 min (3000 rpm), and sera were separated into 1.5 ml micro tubes and then placed in freezer (−20°C). Serum samples were tested for leptin, insulin, and progesterone by ELISA method. Standard commercial kits were used for analysis, and the procedures were adopted as recommended by the manufacturer of these kits.

2.6 Statistical analyses

Data were analyzed as a completely randomized design in factorial arrangement (2 × 2) by using the mixed model procedure of SAS software [19] with fixed effects of treatment and random effects of lamb nested in treatments:

$$Yik = \mu + Di + Lk(Di) + \varepsilon ik \quad (1)$$

where Yij = dependent variable; μ = mean; Di = fixed effect of dietary treatment i; Lk(Di) = effect of lamb k nested in the dietary treatment; εik = error.

For repeated measure date model:

$$Yijk = \mu + Di + timej + Di \times timej + Lk(Di) + \varepsilon ijk \quad (2)$$

where timej = effect of time j as a fixed effect.

Measurements obtained before administration of dietary treatments were used as covariates. The covariates were removed from the model one at a time, starting with the least significant. Least square means, standard error of means, and P-values are reported. Statistical differences were considered significant when $P < 0.05$ and trends are discussed when $P < 0.01$.

3. Results and discussion

Kurdish ewe is the most popular indigenous dairy breed of sheep in the west of Iran. Its main characteristics are high prolificacy and high milk yield. Considering the high genetic potential of Kurdish sheep, it is important to ensure that appropriate management practices are implemented in these intensive production systems.

3.1 Intake, growth, and puberty

Discussing about the topic of sheep and lamb management over the last 40–50 years traditionally involved sheep management, growth development, and early weaning. In the last 10–20 years, the concept of "intensified feeding or accelerated growth" has become a focus of discussion, and during that time the concept has been applied to research programs and on farm in various ways.

The results of intake and BW that were obtained from ewe lambs pre- and post-weaning are summarized in **Table 2**. Results showed that initial BW was similar between all experimental groups ($P > 0.05$), but ewe lambs fed with HQD would gain faster than ewe lambs fed with LQD in BW. And also accelerated BW during the prepubertal period was achieved in the current study affecting the age of puberty (**Table 3**); this is in agreement with the results of Rosales et al. [20] in ewe lambs. BW includes muscle and fat and thus questions interpretation. An important consideration is that BW per se is simply mass and so encompasses physiological or mechanistic process that would affect the reproductive system [21]. In 2009 and 2010, Kenyon et al. indicated that there is a clear positive relationship between BW and reproductive performance in ewe lambs that aligns with the results of present studies.

Results revealed that the HQD treatment increased DMI, compared with the LQD treatment during pre-weaning period ($P < 0.01$). DMI in L-H group was lower than in H-H group, which is similar to the observations by Aguerre et al. [22]. DMI in H-L group was greater than in L-L group, lambs fed with the HQD in pre-weaning had greater DMI when they were fed with the LQD in post-weaning, and it seems that the increase in DMI let to larger body size. Ewe lambs from the H-L treatments also experienced reduced growth rates during post-weaning period, possible reasons for this result may be the larger body size, higher basal metabolism, higher energy, and protein requirements; with regard to rumen capacity and appetite of lambs, the LQD could not cover their needs at period post-weaning. Animals of L-H treatment could respond to diet quality changes but with lower rates than before weaning. Feeding LQD reduces the weight gain of growing animals and can result in greater growth rate once dietary conditions improve, and current results are in agreement with those reported by Drouillard et al. (1991).

Ewe lamb fresh milk intake and milk ME and CP intake were not affected by diet quality among treatments ($P > 0.05$, **Table 2**). During the post-weaning period, lambs of H-H treatment had higher ($P < 0.01$; **Table 2**) DMI, ME, and CP intake compared with other lamb treatments ($P > 0.05$).

The rates of ADG are shown in **Table 2**, indicating differences in the timing of responses to diet quality. Hence, responses to HQD were much greater at a younger

Item	Pre-weaning treatments		Item	Post-weaning treatments			
	HQD	LQD		HQD		LQD	
				H-H	H-L	L-H	L-L
n	20	20	n	10	10	10	10
Intake			**Intake**				
DM (kg/d)	0.97	0.64	DM (kg/day)	1.54	1.21	1.31	0.87
Fresh milk (kg/d)	1.11	1.18	ME (Mcal/day)	3.85	2.42	3.27	1.76
ME (diet + milk, Mcal/d)	3.49	2.44	CP (g/day)	228	104	194	76
CP (diet + milk, g/d)	187.4	103	Puberty age (day)	123	254	168	267
BW			**BW**				
30 days (kg)	10.1	10.2					
120 days (kg)	31.2	22.5	210 days (kg)	43.8	33.9	36.3	26.6
ADG 30–120 days (g/day)	235	136	ADG 121–210 days (g/days)	138	31	153	57
FCR (%)	4.13	4.69	FCR (%)	11.1	38.7	8.57	15.26

Pre-weaning treatments: HQD, high-quality diet; LQD, low-quality diet. Post-weaning treatments: H-H, HQD pre- and post-weaning; H-L, HQD pre-weaning and LQD post-weaning; L-H, LQD pre-weaning and HQD post-weaning; L-L, LQD pre- and post-weaning (control).
DM, dry matter; ME, metabolite energy; CP, crude protein; BW, body weight; ADG, average daily gain; and FCR, feed conversion ratio.

Table 2.
Effects of pre- and post-weaning diet quality on intake and body weight of ewe lambs (30–210 days of age).

age, while responses to HQD were greater for ewe lambs that fed with LQD at pre-weaning and then received HQD at post-weaning, which is in agreement with other studies on sheep and cattle [23–25]. These authors indicate that increased severity of feed restriction is likely to increase the rate of growth after realimentation. Animals fed with HQD had higher BW and ADG compared with animals fed with LQD at pre-weaning period ($P < 0.01$). Lambs on the L-H group during the post-weaning had higher ADG than lambs on H-L and L-L groups ($P < 0.01$). However, lambs had higher ADG than H-H group, but this difference was not significant (153 vs. 138 g/day).

Growth rate and feed conversion ratio (FCR) are considered key production parameters by sheep farmers. Optimizing these parameters can better farm income by improving the production of the farm and/or by improving production efficiency (lambs produced per unit of feed consumed). Lambs consuming the HQD in pre-weaning had similar FCR with lambs fed with the LQD. Ewe lambs consuming the HQD in pre-weaning and LQD in post-weaning (H-L group) had greater FCR than other groups (**Table 2**). Ewe lambs in L-H group had lowest FCR and greater feed efficiency than H-H group.

Nutrition is a factor that influences the start of lamb's puberty and has an important effect on sexual maturity [9]. Most Kurdish ewe lambs achieved puberty by 210–240 days of age when their average live weight was approximately 35 kg or approximately 65% of their estimated mature live weight [26]. The average puberty age of H-H and L-H groups was lower than H-L and L-L groups, respectively ($P < 0.05$, **Table 2**). Based on the results of current study, ewe lambs with higher growth rate were more likely to achieve puberty. And also these lambs were heavier at weaning time and grew faster during the post-weaning period. The ewe lambs of H-L group were heavier than ewe lambs of L-L group at weaning time and post-weaning period. These results are consistent with previous reports that faster growth results in more ewes achieving puberty at a younger age in female sheep [20]. Most of the ewe lambs of L-L group did not show puberty at 210 days of age, and therefore they were removed from the first reproduction table. The average puberty age of H-H sequence was lower than other treatments, with no significant interaction of per- and post-weaning ($P < 0.05$).

3.2 Hormones

The mean of serum insulin and leptin concentrations of ewe lambs at pre- and post-weaning is shown in **Table 3**. Serum insulin concentrations was higher for lambs fed with HQD compared with lambs fed with LQD (4.45 vs. 2.09 μIU/ml, respectively, **Table 3**). Animals in H-H treatments had higher serum insulin concentration at 210 days of age compared with other treatments, while leptin concentration of ewe lambs of L-H group was higher than in other treatments at 210 days of age. These results indicated that maybe increasing weight gain at post-weaning contributed with higher fat fraction and also ultrasonography evidence from fat and muscle diameter of between 12- and 13-rib area support these results (the results were not reported).

Little is known about the importance of leptin in the early postnatal period, despite its potential role in important processes such as mammary gland and appetite regulation and a variety of other effects in the body [21]. Leptin is synthesized and secreted primarily particularly in adipose tissue, in addition to multiple other sites of production including the mammary gland and leptin regulated by multiple hormones including somatotropin, insulin, and IGF-I [27]. Leptin concentration was positively associated with higher values for growth and fat accumulation and therefore with an improvement in reproductive performance [20]. The current results support this concept because leptin concentration was positively correlated with body fat; however, endocrine links to the reproductive control centers have not been clearly identified.

The hormones insulin and leptin have primary roles in the control of reproduction in sheep. In times of decreased feeding, these hormones interact at the hypothalamus to reduce reproduction and enhance feeding [1]. Thus, nutrient reprioritization occurs in part at the expense of reproductive function as a survival mechanism. For example, reduced insulin occurs to spare glucose for central nervous system function, and reduced leptin occurs to allow stimulation of neuropeptide Y to in turn increase appetite as well as changes in anabolic hormones and,

Item	Pre-weaning treatments		Post-weaning treatments			
	HQD	LQD	HQD		LQD	
			H-H	H-L	L-H	L-L
n	20	20	10	10	10	10
Insulin (μIU/ml)	4.45	2.09	4.48	2.32	3.59	1.35
Leptin (ng/ml)	2.84	2.20	3.03	2.06	3.66	1.98
Progesterone (ng/ml)	1.38	0.76	2.98	1.85	2.42	0.95

Pre-weaning treatments: HQD, high-quality diet; LQD, low-quality diet. Post-weaning treatments: H-H, HQD pre- and post-weaning; H-L, HQD pre-weaning and LQD post-weaning; L-H, LQD pre-weaning and HQD post-weaning; L-L, LQD pre- and post-weaning (control).

Table 3.
Effects of pre- and post-weaning diet quality on serum insulin and leptin concentrations of ewe lambs (30–210 days of age).

Item	Pre-weaning treatments		Post-weaning treatments			
	HQD	LQD	HQD		LQD	
			H-H	H-L	L-H	L-L
n	20	20	10	10	10	10
Tail measures (cm)						
Tail length	30.95	27.15	38.00^{a}	33.10^{b}	36.00^{ab}	29.26^{c}
Tail width	27.75	24.55	35.45^{a}	31.34^{b}	32.37^{ab}	27.18^{c}
Tail circumference	56.75^{a}	47.45^{b}	67.24^{a}	55.82^{b}	59.16^{b}	49.52^{c}

^{a,b,c} *Means with distinct subscripts in the same row differ (P < 0.05). Pre-weaning treatments: HQD, high-quality diet; LQD, low-quality diet. Post-weaning treatments: H-H, HQD pre- and post-weaning; H-L, HQD pre-weaning and LQD post-weaning; L-H, LQD pre-weaning and HQD post-weaning; L-L, LQD pre- and post-weaning (control).*

Table 4.
Effects of pre- and post-weaning diet quality on tail measures of ewe lambs (30–210 days of age).

ultimately, reduce Kp and GnRH until feed is more readily available [21]. Rosales et al. [20] reported that leptin levels positively correlated with earlier puberty onset in ewe lambs. And also these authors reported that leptin concentration was not related to age at first estrus, but puberty and BW at first estrus were positively correlated with leptin concentration [20, 28, 29].

Progesterone can be used to monitor the pregnancy status and timing of puberty [30]. Within the post-weaning, serum progesterone concentrations were greater for ewe lambs fed at H-H group than for those fed the L-H, H-L, and L-L treatments, respectively (P < 0.05, **Table 3**). In conclusion, it was concluded that prepubertal plan plays an important role in secretion of progesterone, which leads to early sexual puberty. The present findings demonstrate that in the female lamb, LQD may impair the systems governing the luteinizing hormone that controls follicle growth and cycle hormone (progesterone secretion) and delays puberty.

3.3 Tail measures

At the 120 days of age, HQD lambs had higher tail circumference (P < 0.01; **Table 4**), than LQD lambs. At 210 days of age, after a period of feed restriction of H-L treatment, the average tail length, tail width, and tail circumference of lambs in the H-L group were lower than H-H lambs (P < 0.05; **Table 4**) but showed no difference compared with that of the L-H group (P > 0.05; **Table 4**). Animal growth has been defined as the net accretion of protein and fat in respective tissues, controlled by nutrition, environment, and genetic capacity to grow [31]. Hamouda and Atti [32] revealed that in young lambs, carcass adiposity and particularly fat tail reduce Barbarine meat value as the lamb grows. And also, fat stored in the body is an important energy source when food is rare. In the present work, results showed that better diet with greater energy and protein complementation was able to improve intake and growth performance.

4. Conclusions

The present study confirmed that a HQD improved the BW and ADG at weaning and breeding time. Based on the results of this research, weaning weight, previous nutrition plan, and current nutrition level are factors that determine puberty age, hormone concentration, and tail measures. To conclude, it was concluded that prepubertal plan plays an important role in secretion of progesterone, insulin, and leptin, which can lead to early sexual puberty. And also these strategic plans should improve economic traits at the start of lamb's puberty in sheep husbandry.

Acknowledgements

The authors would like to acknowledge the Nomadic Management Department of Ilam Province (Iran) for providing research opportunities and for their help and collaborations in this work.

Author details

Sedigheh Menatian[1*], Hamidreza Mirzaei Alamouti[2], Farshid Fatahnia[1] and Reza Masoumi[2]

1 Department of Animal Science, Faculty of Agriculture, Ilam University, Ilam, Iran

2 Department of Animal Science, Faculty of Agriculture, Zanjan University, Zanjan, Iran

*Address all correspondence to: menatian@alumni.znu.ac.ir

References

[1] Besson M, Aubin J, Komen H, Poelman M, Quillet E, Vandeputte M, et al. Environmental impacts of genetic improvement of growth rate and feed conversion ratio in fish farming under rearing density and nitrogen output limitations. Journal of Cleaner Production. 2016;**116**:100-109

[2] Rosa HJD, Bryant MJ. Seasonality of reproduction in sheep. Small Ruminant Research. 2003;**48**:155-171

[3] Kenyon PR, Thompson AN, Morris ST. Breeding ewe lambs successfully to improve lifetime performance. Small Ruminant Research. 2014;**118**:2-15

[4] Young JM, Thompson AN, Kennedy AJ. Bio economic modeling to identify the relative importance of a range of critical control points for prime lamb production systems in south-west Victoria. Animal Production Science. 2010;**50**:748-756

[5] Kenyon PR, van der Linden DS, West DM, Morris ST. The effect of breeding hoggets on lifetime performance. New Zealand Journal of Agricultural Research. 2011;**54**:321-330

[6] Ettema JF, Santos JEP. Impact of age at calving on lactation, reproduction, health, and income in first-parity Holsteins on commercial farms. Journal of Dairy Science. 2004;**87**:2730-2742

[7] Umberger SH. The effect of accelerated growth and fattening from early weaning to parturition on ewe reproduction and lactation [PhD thesis]. Raleigh: North Carolina State University; 1980

[8] Wallace J, Bourke D, Da Silva P, Aitken R. Nutrient partitioning during adolescent pregnancy. Reproduction. 2001;**122**:347-357

[9] HernandezF,ElviraL,Gonzalez-MartinJV, Gonzalez-Bulnes A, Astiz S. Influence of age at first lambing on reproductive and productive performance of Lacaune dairy sheep under an intensive management system. The Journal of Dairy Research. 2011;**78**:160-167

[10] Downing J, Lees JL. Unpublished data cited by J.L. Lees in a paper read at the British Council Course No. 729. Edinburgh, March 1978; 1977

[11] Mulvaney FJ, Morris ST, Kenyon PR, West DM, Morel PCH. Effect of live weight at the start of the breeding period and live weight gain during the breeding period and pregnancy on reproductive performance of hoggets and the live weight of their lambs. New Zealand Journal of Agricultural Research. 2010;**53**:355-364

[12] Dyrmundsson OR. Natural factors affecting puberty and reproductive performance in ewe lambs: A review. Livestock Production Science. 1981;**8**:55-65

[13] NRC. Nutrient Requirements of Small Ruminants: Sheep, Goats. Washington, DC: National Academies Press; 2007

[14] AOAC. Official Methods of Analysis. 16th ed. Washington, DC: Association of Official Analytical Chemists; 1995

[15] Van Soest PJ, Robertson JB, Lew BA. Methods for dietary fiber, neutral detergent fiber, and nonstarch polysaccharides in relation to animal nutrition. Journal of Dairy Science. 1991;**74**:3583-3597

[16] NRC. Nutrient Requirements of Dairy Cattle. 7th ed. Washington, DC: National Academies Press; 2001

[17] Van der Linden DS, Lopez-Villalobos N, Kenyon PR, Thorstensen E, Jenkinson CMC,

Peterson SW, et al. Comparison of four techniques to estimate milk production in singleton-rearing non-dairy ewes. Small Ruminant Research. 2010;**90**:18-26

[18] Treacher TT, Caja G. Nutrition during lactation. In: Freer MH, Dove H, editors. Sheep Nutrition. Australia: CSIRO Publishing; 2002

[19] SAS Institute. SAS®/STAT Software, Release 8.0. Cary, NC, USA: SAS Institute, Inc.; 2003

[20] Rosales Nieto CA, Ferguson MB, Macleay CA, Briegel JR, Wood DA, Martin GB, et al. Ewe lambs with higher breeding values for growth achieve higher reproductive performance when mated at age 8 months. Theriogenology. 2013;**80**:427-435

[21] Daniel JA, Foradori CD, Whitlock BK, Sartin JL. Hypothalamic integration of nutrient status and reproduction in the sheep. Reprod. Dom. Anim. 2013;**48**(Suppl. 1):44-52

[22] Aguerre M, Cajarville C, Kozloski JV, Repetto GL. Intake and digestive responses by ruminants fed fresh temperate pasture supplemented with increased levels of sorghum grain: A comparison between cattle and sheep. Animal Feed Science and Technology. 2013;**186**:12-19

[23] Abouheif M, Al-Owaimer A, Kraidees M, Metwally H, Shafey T. Effect of restricted feeding and realimentation on feed performance and carcass characteristic of growing lambs. Rev. Bras. Zootecn. 2013;**42**:95-101

[24] Drouillard JS, Ferrell CL, Klopfenstein TJ, Britton RA. Compensatory growth following metabolizable protein or energy restrictions in beef steers. Journal of Animal Science. 1991;**69**:811-818

[25] Yang J, Hou X, Gao A, Wang H. Effect of dietary energy and protein restriction followed by realimentation on pituitary mRNA expression of growth hormone and related genes in lambs. Small Ruminant Research. 2014;**119**:39-44

[26] Ehtesham SH, Vakili AR. The effect of spent mushroom substrate on blood metabolites and weight gain in Kurdish male lambs. Entomology and Applied Science Letters. 2015;**2**(1):29-33

[27] Smith JL, Sheffield LG. Production and regulation of leptin in bovine mammary epithelial cells. Domestic Animal Endocrinology. 2002;**2**:145-155

[28] Kenyon PR, Smith SL, Morel PCH, Morris ST, West DM. The effect of the maturity and prior breeding activity of rams and body condition score of ewe hoggets on the reproductive performance of ewe hoggets. New Zealand Veterinary Journal. 2009;**57**:290-294

[29] Kenyon PR, Morris ST, West DM. Proportion of rams and the condition of ewe lambs at joining influences their breeding performance. Animal Production Science. 2010;**50**:454-459

[30] Olfati A, Moghaddam GH, Moradi Kor N, Bakhtiari M. The relationship between progesterone and biochemical constituents of amniotic fluid with placenta traits in Iranian crossbred ewes (Arkhar-merino × Ghezel). Asian Pacific Journal of Tropical Medicine. 2014;**7**(Suppl 1):162-166

[31] MacGheea ME, Bradleya JS, McCoski SR, Reeg AM, Ealy AD, Johnson SE. Plane of nutrition affects growth rate, organ size and skeletal muscle satellite cell activity in newborn calves. Journal of Animal Physiology and Animal Nutrition. 2016;**42**:1-9

[32] Hamouda MB, Atti N. Comparison growth curves of lamb fat tail measurements and their relationship with body weight in Babarine sheep. Small Ruminant Research. 2011;**95**:120-127

Chapter 4

Bioclimatic Influence on the Pregnancy Rate in Embryo-Recipient Cows in the Amazonian Biome

Jefferson Viana Alves Diniz, Laine Oliveira da Silva, Marina Marie Bento Nogueira, Rosano Ramos de Freitas, Marcos Nereu Luckner, Rafael Augusto Satrapa, José Antonio Dell'Aqua Junior and Eunice Oba

Abstract

The objective of the research was to evaluate the effect of the climate, through the parameters of rectal temperature (RT), temperature and humidity index (THI), and plasma cortisol concentration, on the physiological responses of embryo-recipient cows in the Amazonian biome. For the conduction of the experiment in which 11 rural properties participated, 235 crossbred cows were used as embryo recipients. The embryos were obtained by means of the in vitro production technique (PIV). The recipients were divided into batches and submitted based on the simplification of the P36 protocol for fixed-time embryo transfer (FTET). To the day of embryo transfer, blood samples were collected by venipuncture of the coccygeal vein in tubes with anticoagulant. Plasma cortisol dosages were done by solid-phase radioimmunoassay (RIA) technique using commercial kits. The rectal temperature of each of the recipients submitted to the protocol was verified using a digital clinical thermometer, and the ambient temperature and the relative humidity of the air were evaluated in this moment, both with the aid of own digital equipment. Statistical analysis of the parameters evaluated was Pearson's correlation and Student's t-test at a significance level of 5%. In the analysis of variance, it was observed that there was a significant difference in plasma cortisol and THI among the groups, where lower mean values were found in the GP group. The Amazonian climate is an inducer of thermal stress, which can cause abnormalities in the estral cycle and changes in the synthesis of sex hormones and embryonic development and, consequently, negatively affect the pregnancy rate in embryo-recipient cows, even in races more adapted to the tropics, as demonstrated by the RT, THI, and plasma cortisol parameters.

Keywords: embryo transfer, thermal stress, thermoregulation, THI

1. Introduction

Brazil is a predominantly tropical country, with high average temperatures during the year, generally causing thermal stress to the production animals and causing physiological imbalances that, in turn, cause an increase in the net energy requirements for maintenance, which, consequently, causes a decrease in the available energy for the productive processes [1]. The heat stress condition harms homeostasis and promotes endocrine changes that have negative effects on reproductive events in the bovine female [2].

The stressor agent, through the preoptic area of the central nervous system, acts on the neurosecretory cells of the paraventricular nucleus of the hypothalamus, and, from this stimulation, these cells produce the corticotrophin-releasing hormone (CRH), which promotes the secretion of the adrenocorticotrophic hormone (ACTH) by the adenohypophysis [3]. ACTH acts on the adrenal glands stimulating the secretion of corticosteroids, such as the hormone cortisol [4]. Thus, cows undergoing thermal stress stimulate with greater intensity the hypothalamic-pituitary-adrenal axis, increasing the concentrations of ACTH and cortisol [5]. This hormone interferes with mechanisms related to fertility, such as resumption of estrous cycle, ovulation of a competent oocyte, and establishment of gestation [6].

However, for a long time, in trying to overcome barriers, we have sought the support of reproductive biotechnologies with a view to increasing production, through the use of techniques such as artificial insemination (AI), artificial insemination at fixed time (AIFT), and fertilization in vitro [7, 8]. Brazil has a great representation in the world scenario of in vitro embryo production, and this is mainly due to the work done with zebu breeds with which best results are obtained, probably due to their better adaptation to the tropics [9]. In this sense, the objective of the research was to evaluate the effect of the climate, through the parameters of rectal temperature (RT), temperature and humidity index (THI), and plasma cortisol concentration, on the physiological responses of embryo-recipient cows in the Amazonian biome.

2. Material and methods

The study was elaborated according to the ethics committee of the Faculdade de Medicina Veterinária e Zootecnia—Universidade Estadual Paulista Júlio de Mesquita Filho (case number 227/2011). For the conduction of the experiment in which 11 rural properties participated, distributed in 6 municipalities of the state of Acre (9°6′36″ S, 70°31′12″ W), 235 crossbred cows were used as embryo recipients (*Bos taurus taurus* × *Bos taurus indicus*), native of Acre, uni- or multiparous, aged between 3 and 6 years, non-lactating, raised in an extensive regime, with water and mineral salt ad libitum, and with body condition score between 3 and 4, on a scale of 1–5 [10].

The embryos were obtained by means of the in vitro production technique (PIV), using semen and oocytes from selected Gir dairy cattle. The recipients were divided into batches containing 10–12 animals and submitted to the same estrus induction/synchronization protocol. Based on the simplification of the P36 protocol for fixed-time embryo transfer (FTET) described by [11], the protocols were developed as follows: on a random day of the estrous cycle (D0), each of the recipients received 1 g of P4 by an intravaginal device and 2.5 mg of estradiol benzoate (EB) intramuscularly (IM). On the eighth day (D8), the P4 device was withdrawn, and 150 μg of D-cloprostenol (PGF2α), 400 IU of eCG, and 1 mg of BE were given intramuscularly. On the 16th day (D16), each recipient received a transferred embryo (blastocyst, grade 1 or 2) after being previously diagnosed by ultrasound of a corpus luteum (LC) in one of the ovaries. On the 41st day (D41), the diagnosis of gestation (DG) was made.

Concomitantly to the day of embryo transfer, blood samples were collected by venipuncture of the coccygeal vein in tubes with anticoagulant. The obtained plasma was fractionated in 1.5 mL microtubes duly identified and stored at 20°C negative until sent to the laboratory for analysis. Plasma cortisol dosages were done by solid-phase radioimmunoassay (RIA) technique using commercial kits.

Prior to performing at the D16 ultrasonography evaluation, the rectal temperature of each of the recipients submitted to the protocol was verified using a digital clinical thermometer, and the ambient temperature and the relative humidity of the air were evaluated in this moment, both with the aid of own digital equipment. The temperature and humidity index was calculated according to [12], using the formula

$$\text{THI} = 0.8\,\text{Tbs} + \text{RH}\frac{\text{Tbs} - 14.3}{100} + 46.3$$

where Tbs refers to the dry-bulb temperature (°C) and RH to relative humidity (%). Statistical analysis of the parameters evaluated was Pearson's correlation and Student's t-test at a significance level of 5%.

3. Results

The rates of yield of the embryo recipients and of pregnancy after application of the protocol were 67.23 (158/235) and 34.18% (54/158), respectively. Regarding the ambient temperature (RT), the relative air humidity (RH), and the RT recorded during the 15 months of the survey, mean values are 30.07, 69.23, and 39.28°C, respectively.

It was found that there was a significant difference of the THI and RT between the two established groups: pregnant cows (GP) and nonpregnant cows (GNP), where the lowest mean values were found in the GP group. It was also found that both groups had a significant and positive correlation between the THI and RT parameters (**Table 1**).

The climatic variables in this study refer to the typical days of the Amazon region, collected on nonconsecutive dates. It was verified that the GNP group for the THI parameter (81.83 ± 0.03) had values above the care range; the GP group presented values below the safety range. It was also found that the THI values (70.50 ± 0.10) of the GP group were below the established values of 72–78.

Parameters	GNP	GP
THI	81.83 ± 0.03^a	70.50 ± 0.10^b
RT(°C)	39.52 ± 0.24^a	38.66 ± 0.28^b
Pearson correlation between the THI and RT	(r = 0.73; p = 0.0208)	(r = 0.85; p = 0.0126)

GNP, not pregnant group; GP, pregnant group; THI, temperature and humidity index; RT, rectal temperature. Distinct lowercase letters on the same line indicate significant differences by the Student's t-test at the 5% level of significance.

Table 1.
Correlation between THI and RT (average ± standard error) in the groups which are not pregnant and pregnant.

Parameters	GNP	GP
Cortisol (ng/mL)	17.78 ± 5.54^a	13.78 ± 4.74^b
THI	81.83 ± 0.03^a	70.50 ± 0.10^b
Pearson correlation between the cortisol and THI	(r = 0.45; p = 0.0368)	(r = 0.76; p = 0.0186)

GNP, not pregnant group; GP, pregnant group; THI, temperature and humidity index. Distinct lowercase letters on the same line indicate significant differences by the Student's t-test at the 5% level of significance.

Table 2.
Correlation between plasma cortisol concentrations and THI (average ± standard error) in the groups which are not pregnant and pregnant.

In the analysis of variance, it was observed that there was a significant difference in plasma cortisol and THI among the groups, where lower mean values were found in the GP group. It was also found that both groups had a significant and positive correlation between cortisol and THI parameters (**Table 2**).

4. Discussion

On the yield of protocols, similar results have been reported by [13, 14], with rates of 72.9 and 65%, respectively. The results for pregnancy rate were also shown to be close to those described by [15], which reached 36.60% (108/295), using eCG in D8.

The mean value of the recorded RT was attested as higher than the maximum of 39.1°C, as mentioned by [16], also remaining outside the limits of normality described by [17]. On the other hand, [18] state that cattle of all races have an average rectal temperature of 38.3°C with some variations. However, the RT remained within the physiological values that according to [19] for adult cattle is between 37.5 and 39.3°C. Therefore, the RT of the NP group exceeded the thermoneutral zone in which the maintenance of homeothermia occurs with a maximum mobilization of the mechanisms of heat dissipation, responsible for thermoregulation, and this deviation of energy may be responsible for a decrease in reproductive performance.

The comfort zone for cattle is relatively small, whereas for the European breeds, it is between −1 and 16°C and for the zebu breeds between 10 and 27°C [20], with limit critical from 35°C [21, 22]. In other words, the high-temperature indices of the Amazon region present a great challenge to the animals, requiring them to develop adaptive mechanisms for heat dissipation. However, the temperature range that confers thermal comfort in which there is minimum energy expenditure to maintain the homeothermia also depends on the relative humidity of the air [1].

The animals of this experiment were found in the Amazon biome characterized by high temperature and humidity [21, 22]. Therefore, when the air humidity is low, evaporation is facilitated; otherwise the evaporation process becomes slow or even null, making maintenance of homeothermia difficult [23]. Thus, these conditions of heat and relative air humidity, almost always, are above the zone of thermal comfort for the animals, demanding, by them, energy expenditure in terms of thermoregulatory physiological mechanisms in the attempt of heat dissipation [24]. However, there are occasions in which the loss of body heat becomes ineffective, and then thermal stress of the animal occurs, which is often a limiting factor for development, production, and reproduction [25].

The reproductive efficiency of dairy cattle exposed to adverse climatic conditions is compromised when temperature and humidity are high and solar radiation is intense for most of the year [26], a recurrent situation in the Amazonian biome.

In the case of the use of PIV, embryo development becomes impaired when cows suffer from heat stress on AI day or up to 7 days after the procedure, which leads to less embryonic viability [2], which may render the results of the technique unfeasible.

In a study with Dutch cows by Martello et al. [19], THI values up to 74 correspond to the safety range and from 74 to 78 care range. Igono et al. [27], however, consider THI above 76 in any environment stressful for cows with high milk yield. The climatic variables presented in this study indicate mild thermal stress; thus, the highest values of THI found in the GNP group indicate an environmental situation favoring stress for the animals, where the thermal condition was above that considered comfort. These processes may cause reproductive performance below ideal, such as a decrease in conception rate during the hot season by 20–30% [28] and significant economic losses [29]. Climatic conditions may be an important contributor to the low fertility of dairy cows during the summer months, especially in high-yielding cows [30].

Plasma concentrations of cortisol, above 10 ng/mL for zebu breeds, were similar to those reported by [31] for both groups. Therefore, because it is considered the stress hormone, its evaluation, although expensive, has become of great value for the establishment of the animal welfare condition [32]. Higher production of cortisol causes negative feedback in the hypothalamus, decreasing the synthesis of gonadotrophin-releasing hormone (GnRH), and consequently reduces the release of gonadotrophins FSH and LH, facts that, in the end, are responsible for the low production of the gonadal hormones [33]. The reduction of the latter, in turn, causes less manifestation of estrus, low conception rate, embryonic mortality, and abortions [34].

The lower plasma cortisol concentration in the GP group possibly favored the embryonic quality and maintenance of gestation in relation to the GNP group. Garcia-Ispierto et al. [35] found that the probability of pregnancy loss increases by 1.05 times each unit increase in THI between days 21 and 30 gestations. Due to the results obtained, it is possible to observe that the animals of the GNP group were in a situation of thermal stress, due to the increase of the reported plasma cortisol and of the THI that can act negatively on the luteal function, consequently, and thus the maintenance and recognition of pregnancy [36].

Embryonic development is very susceptible to thermal stress, especially on the third day of development, reducing the proportion of embryos that continue to evolve [37]. In addition, the reduction of embryonic growth is associated with lower levels of interferon-tau that acts on the inhibition of pulsatile secretion of prostaglandin F2α, that is, low levels of interferon-tau may not block the regression of the corpus luteum, making it difficult to maintain the gestation [35]; thus, animals that are under thermal stress are likely to present alterations in the embryonic production of interferon-tau, which causes losses in the maintenance of gestation. Therefore, the techniques used in breeding should be associated with measures that reduce the effects of the thermal environment on production animals [38].

5. Conclusion

The Amazonian climate is an inducer of thermal stress, which can cause abnormalities in the estral cycle and changes in the synthesis of sex hormones and embryonic development and, consequently, negatively affect the pregnancy rate in embryo-recipient cows, even in races more adapted to the tropics, as demonstrated by the RT, THI, and plasma cortisol parameters. Therefore, it is recommended to adopt measures that may reduce the effect of environmental conditions on the reproductive performance of production animals.

Author details

Jefferson Viana Alves Diniz[1*], Laine Oliveira da Silva[2], Marina Marie Bento Nogueira[2], Rosano Ramos de Freitas[2], Marcos Nereu Luckner[2], Rafael Augusto Satrapa[2], José Antonio Dell'Aqua Junior[3] and Eunice Oba[3]

1 Instituto Federal do Acre—IFAC, Sena Madureira, AC, Brasil

2 Universidade Federal do Acre—UFAC, Rio Branco, AC, Brasil

3 Universidade Estadual Paulista Júlio de Mesquita Filho, Botucatu, SP, Brasil

*Address all correspondence to: jefferson.diniz@ifac.edu.br

References

[1] Silva RG. Introdução a Bioclimatologia Animal. São Paulo: Nobel; 2000

[2] Macedo GG, Costa e Silva EV, Pinho RO, Assumpção TI, Jacomini JO, Santos RM, et al. O estresse por calor diminui a fertilidade de fêmeas bovinas por afetar o desenvolvimento oocitário e o embrionário. Revista Brasileira de Reprodução Animal. 2014;**38**:80-85

[3] Minton JE. Function of the hypothalamic-pituitary-adrenal axis and the sympathetic nervous system in models of acute stress in domestic farm animals. Journal of Animal Science. 1994;**72**:1891-1898

[4] Breen KM, Billings HJ, Wagenmaker ER, Wessinger EW, Karsch FJ. Endocrine basis for disruptive effect of cortisol on preovulatory events. Endocrinology. 2005;**146**:2107-2115

[5] Cooke RF, Arthington JD, Araujo DB, Lamb GC. Effects of acclimation to human interaction on performance, temperament, physiological responses, and pregnancy rates of Brahman-crossbred cows. Journal of Animal Science. 2009;**87**:4125-4132

[6] Dobson H, Tebble JE, Smith RF. Is stress really all that important? Theriogenology. 2001;**55**:65-73

[7] Baruselli PS, Reis EL, Marques MO, Nasser LF, Bó GA. The use of hormonal treatments to improve reproductive performance of anestrous beef cattle in tropical climates. Animal Reproduction Science. 2004;**82-83**:479-486

[8] Vieira RJ. Biotécnicas aplicadas à reprodução bovina: Generalidades. Revista Acadêmica Ciência Animal. 2012;**22**:55-65

[9] Viana JHM, Siqueira LG, Palhao MP, Camargo LS. Use of in vitro fertilization technique in the last decade and its effect on Brazilian embryo industry and animal production. Acta Scientiae Veterinariae. 2010;**38**:661-674

[10] Ferreira AM, Torres CAA. Perda de peso corporal e cessação da atividade ovariana luteínica cíclica em vacas mestiças leiteiras. Pesquisa Agropecuária Brasileira. 1993;**28**:411-418

[11] Barros CM, Nogueira MFG. Embryo transfer in *Bos indicus* cattle. Theriogenology. 2001;**56**:1483-1496

[12] Pires MFA, Ferreira AM, Saturnino HM, Teodoro RL. Taxa de gestação em fêmeas da raça Holandesa confinadas em free stall, no verão e inverno. Arquivo Brasileiro de Medicina Veterinária e Zootecnia. 2002;**54**:57-63

[13] Barreiros TRR, Blaschi W, Borsato EA, Ludwig HÊ, Silva DRM, Seneda MM. Comparação das taxas de prenhez entre receptoras com corpos lúteos cavitários ou compactos após protocolo de sincronização com cloprostenol ou transferência de embriões em tempo fixo. Semina: Ciências Agrárias. 2006;**27**:657-664

[14] Rodrigues CA, Ranieri AL, Teixeira AA, Vieira LM, Ferreira RM, Ayres H, et al. Eficiência reprodutiva de receptoras holandesas de alta produção sincronizadas para TETF com protocolos com ou sem estradiol e/ou eCG. In: XXIV Reunião anual da sociedade brasileira de tecnologia de embriões; Porto de Galinhas; 2010

[15] Baruselli PS, Ferreira RM, Sá FIlho MF, Nasser LFT, Rodrigues CA, Bó GA. Bovine embryo transfer recipient synchronization and management in tropical environments. Reproduction, Fertility, and Development. 2010;**22**:67-74

[16] Dukes HH, Swenson MJ. Fisiologia dos Animais Domésticos. 12th ed. Rio de Janeiro: Guanabara Koogan; 2006

[17] Robinson EN. Termorregulação. In: Cunningham JG, editor. Tratado de fisiologia veterinária. 2th ed. Rio de Janeiro: Guanabara Koogan; 1999

[18] McDowell RE, Lee DHK, Fohrman MH. The measurement of water evaporation from limited areas of a normal body surface. Journal of Animal Science. 1954;**13**:405-416

[19] Martello LS, Peixoto AP, Regis JEF, Nascimento JWB, Araujo TGP, Lisboa ACC. Respostas fisiológicas e produtivas de vacas holandesas em lactação submetidas a diferentes ambientes. Revista Brasileira de Zootecnia. 2004;**33**:181-191

[20] Santos SA, McManus C, Souza GS, Soriano BMA, Silva RAMS, Comastri Filho JA, et al. Variações da temperatura corporal e da pele de vacas e bezerros das raças Pantaneira e Nelore no Pantanal. Archivos de Zootecnia. 2005;**54**:237-244

[21] Azevedo M, Pires MFA, Saturnino HM, Lana AMQ, Sampaio IBM, Monteiro JBN, et al. Estimativa de níveis críticos superiores do índice de temperatura e umidade para vacas leiteiras 1/2, 3/4 e 7/8 Holandês-zebu em lactação. Revista Brasileira de Zootecnia. 2005;**34**:2000-2008

[22] Furtado DA, Peixoto AP, Regis JEF, Nascimento JWB, Araujo TGP, Lisboa ACC. Termorregulação e desempenho de tourinhos Sindi e Guzerá, no agreste paraibano. Revista Brasileira de Engenharia Agrícola e Ambiental. 2012;**16**:1022-1028

[23] Wilson DCS, Corbett AD, Bovell DL. A preliminary study of the short circuit current (Isc) responses of sweat gland cells from normal and anhidrotic horses to purinergic and adrenergic agonists. Journal Compilation. 2007;**18**:152-160

[24] Baêta FC, Souza C. Ambiência em edificações rurais: conforto animal. Viçosa: UFV; 1997

[25] Silva RG, Gaudiosi MC. Termólise evaporativa em ovinos sob altas temperaturas. In: anais do Congresso Brasileiro de Biometeorologia; Jaboticabal. 1995. pp. 193-203

[26] Kamal R, Dutt T, Patel M, Dey A, Bharti PK, Chandran PC. Heat stress and effect of shade materials on hormonal and behavior response of dairy cattle: A review. Tropical Animal Health and Production. 2018;**50**:701-706

[27] Igono MO, Bjtvedt G, Sanford-Crane HT. Environmental profile and critical temperature effects on milk production of Holsteins cows in desert climate. International Journal of Biometeorology. 1992;**36**:77-87

[28] De Rensis F, Marconi P, Capelli T, Gatti F, Facciolongo F, Franzini S, et al. Fertility in postpartum dairy cows in winter or summer following estrus synchronization and fixed time AI after the induction of an LH surge with GnRH or hCG. Theriogenology. 2002;**58**:1675-1687

[29] Collier RJ, Dahl GE, Vanbaale MJ. Major advances associated with environmental effects on dairy cattle. Journal of Dairy Science. 2006;**89**:1244-1253

[30] Kadzere CT, Murphy MR, Silanikove N, Maltz E. Heat stress in lactating dairy cows: A review. Livestock Production Science. 2002;**77**:59-91

[31] Yoshida C, Nakao T. Response of plasma cortisol and progesterone after ACTH challenge in ovariectomized lactating dairy cows. Reproduction and Development. 2005;**51**:99-107

[32] Benatti LAT. Avaliação do cortisol, perfil hematológico e proteico na resposta dos bovinos ao estresse. Veterinary Journal. 2010;**159**:201-206

[33] Menezes SRS. Efeitos do clima na performance reprodutiva de bovinos leiteiros nos Açores. Reproduction and Development. 2010;**51**:99-107

[34] Ferro FRA, Cavalcanti Neto CC, Toledo Filho MR, Ferri STS, Montaldo YC. Efeito do estresse calórico no desempenho reprodutivo de vacas leiteiras. Revista Verde. 2010;**5**:01-25

[35] Garcia-Ispierto F, Lopez-Gatius G, Bech-Sabat P. Climate factors affecting conception rate of high producing dairy cows in northeastern Spain. Theriogenology. 2007;**67**:1379-1385

[36] Reis LSLS, Pardo PE, Oba E, Kronka SN, Frazatti-Gallina NM. Matricaria chamomilla CH12 decreases handling stressing Nelore calves. Journal of Veterinary Science. 2006;**7**:189-192

[37] Sartori R, Gumen A, Guenther JN, Souza AH, Caraviello DZ, Willtbank MC. Comparison of artificial insemination versus embryo transfer in lactating dairy cows. Theriogenology. 2006;**65**:1311-1321

[38] Habeeb AAM, Gad AE, El-Tarabany AA, Atta MAA. Negative effects of heat stress on growth and milk production of farm animals. Journal of Animal Husbandry and Dairy Sciences. 2018;**2**:1-12

Chapter 5

Recent Advance in Genome Editing-Based Gene Modification in Pigs

Masahiro Sato, Kazuchika Miyoshi, Hiroaki Kawaguchi, Emi Inada, Issei Saitoh and Akihide Tanimoto

Abstract

Recently, a series of genome editing technologies including ZFNs, TALENs, and CRISPR/Cas9 systems have enabled gene modification in the endogenous target genes of various organisms including pigs, which are important for agricultural and biomedical research. Owing to its simple application for gene knockout and ease of use, the CRISPR/Cas9 is now in common use worldwide. The most important aspect of this process is the selection of the method used to deliver genome editing components to embryos. In earlier stages, zygote microinjection of these components [single guide RNA (sgRNA) + DNA/mRNA for Cas9] into the cytoplasm and/or nuclei of a zygote has been frequently employed. However, this method is always associated with the generation of mosaic embryos in which genome-edited and unedited cells are mixed together. To avoid this mosaic issue, *in vitro* electroporation of zygotes in the presence of sgRNA mixed with Cas9 protein, referred to as a ribonucleoprotein (RNP), is now in frequent use. This review provides a historical background of the production of genome-edited pigs and also presents current research concerning how genome editing is induced in somatic cell nuclear transfer-derived embryos that have been reconstituted with normal nuclei.

Keywords: genome editing, CRISPR/Cas9, ZFNs, TALENs, pigs, gene modification, microinjection, electroporation, somatic cell nuclear transfer, knock out, knock in, gene-engineered, ribonucleoprotein

1. Introduction

The domestic pig has been widely used as a large animal model in biomedical research, as it is similar to humans with respect to the size of body and internal organs, longevity, anatomy, physiology, and metabolic profile [1]. Modification of the porcine genome is also important for studying the mechanisms underlying genetic disorders, developing therapeutic drugs, and improving pig meat production yields [2, 3]. Over the past three decades, attempts have been made to modify the porcine genome using genetic engineering technology, starting after Gordon et al. [4] first reported DNA microinjection (MI)-based production of transgenic (Tg) mice. Hammer et al. [5] first reported the successful production of Tg piglets using the technique reported by Gordon et al. [4], but attaining this result was more difficult than for rodents, where pronuclei are clearly visible using an optical microscope.

In the case of porcine zygotes, pronuclei are difficult to see due to the presence of high lipid content in the cytoplasm. Researchers must briefly centrifuge zygotes to visualize the pronuclei prior to MI [5], which is labor-intensive and requires skill. Moreover, MI-mediated transgene integration into host chromosomes occurs randomly, which often causes gene silencing [6]. However, for precise and efficient genetic modification in the porcine genome, homologous recombination (HR)-based gene targeting technology may be recommended, which was first developed by Smithies' group in mice [7]. In this case, the use of germline-competent embryonic stem (ES) cells is a prerequisite. These ES cells are first transfected with a targeting vector and then recombinant ES clones showing successful targeting are obtained. This vector usually contains a gene of interest (GOI) to be integrated into the target locus, together with a selection marker gene such a neomycin resistance gene (*neo*), and DNA sequences of appropriate length, termed homology arms (HA), that correspond to the endogenous target gene, are placed at both ends of the DNA containing the GOI and a marker gene. Chimeric mice can be obtained through blastocyst injection with the targeted ES clones, and the resulting chimeric mice would contribute to produce heterozygous mice carrying mutated traits (GOI/selection marker gene) in the target locus [8]. Unfortunately, there are no germline-competent porcine ES cells, despite extensive efforts [9–13]. Thus, to date, production of gene-targeted pigs derived from recombinant porcine ES cells has not yet been successful.

In 1996, scientists at *the Roslin Institute* (Wilmut and colleagues) first succeeded in producing cloned sheep using somatic cell nuclear transfer (SCNT) technology. They used fetal fibroblasts [14] or adult mammary gland-derived fibroblasts [15] as SCNT donors. Notably, prior to these reports, an attempt to produce cloned embryos by the similar technique shown by the *Roslin's* group has been made by Prather et al. [16], who performed transfer of nuclei from two, four and eight-cell embryos to the enucleated oocytes and successfully produced one piglets that had been derived from the four-cell embryo's nucleus. This approach is called "blastomere transplantation," which is basically different from the somatic cell-based SCNT. Generally, fibroblasts used as SCNT donors can proliferate actively *in vitro*, and therefore are considered to be ideal cells for transgenesis or gene targeting. If these engineered fibroblasts are used for SCNT, the resulting cloned embryos and piglets should have the engineered traits in their genome. This possibility was first proven by *the scientists at the Roslin Institute* [17, 18] who successfully produced genetically engineered (GE) cloned sheep through SCNT using GE fetal fibroblasts. Since then, SCNT using GE cells as SCNT donors has been a common approach for production of knockout (KO) or Tg piglets [19, 20]. However, as mentioned below, the efficiency of producing cloned GE piglets is extremely low and the preparation of GE donor cells is laborious and time-consuming [21]. During the past two decades, production of only a few GE (KO) piglets has been reported by traditional approaches [22–27]. Moreover, almost all resulting KO piglets were heterozygous with respect to the KO allele, thus requiring additional tasks such as breeding (likely one or two generations), sequence targeting, or *in vitro* cell cloning to obtain homozygous KO animals [28], which is also laborious, expensive, and time-consuming.

However, this situation drastically changed when new gene-targeting technologies emerged for precisely manipulating mammalian genomes, called "second-generation genome editing." These technologies require the design of site-specific engineered nucleases which can be zinc-finger nucleases (ZFNs), transcription activator-like effector nucleases (TALENs) or clustered regularly interspaced short palindromic repeat-associated protein 9 (CRISPR/Cas9) nucleases, all of which induce a double-stranded break (DSB) at a specific site in the genome. This DSB facilitates genetic modification such as nonhomologous end-joining (NHEJ) and homology directed repair (HDR) [29], as described below. Using these genome-editing systems, many

GE piglets have been produced using SCNT of genome-edited cells, or direct microinjection of genome-editing components (including engineered endonucleases) into the cytoplasm of zygotes, as described below in more detail.

2. Background of second-generation genome editing

As mentioned above, site-specific engineered nucleases are used in these genome-editing techniques. ZFNs, TALENs, and CRISPR/Cas9 can all bind to DNA and induce DSB, which triggers endogenous DNA repair. If the template DNA is absent, the DSB is repaired via the NHEJ pathway where insertion or deletion of nucleotides (hereinafter called "indels") can happen in the cleaved area. These indels often cause frameshift of the amino acid sequence, leading to the generation of abnormal proteins or formation of a premature stop codon leading to cessation of protein synthesis. If template DNA homologous to the target site is present, it is inserted into the cleaved area via a site-specific HR event which is called HDR. Generally, NHEJ occurs in cells independent of its cell cycle, but HDR occurs primarily in dividing cells [30].

The ZFN technique uses the ZF protein (which binds to the target DNA) and the endonuclease *Fok* I (which cleaves DNA) [31]. ZF protein has several protein motifs capable of recognizing specific sequences of three nucleotides and binding to them. Notably, Urnov et al. [32] first demonstrated that ZFN is effective to induce DNA editing at the endogenous target gene in mammalian cells. Its targeting efficiency was over 18% in the absence of drug selection, which is ~1000-fold higher than that achieved by traditional gene targeting.

The TALEN technique uses proteins, termed transcription activator-like effectors (TALEs), which contain 33–35 amino acid repeats that flank a central DNA binding region (amino acids 12 and 13), and *Fok* I nuclease, as in ZFN, thus the term TALE nucleases (TALENs) [33–35]. Notably, the design and engineering of TALENs is simpler than that of ZFN, and thus can be done faster [35, 36].

CRISPR/Cas9 employs a short (20 bp) RNA sequence called single-guide RNA (sgRNA) which can bind to the specific chromosomal DNA site together with the Cas9 endonuclease [37–40]. Once bound, two independent nuclease domains in Cas9 each cleave one of the DNA strand's three bases upstream of the protospacer adjacent motif (PAM), introducing DSB at the target site of the host chromosome, which is then repaired by NHEJ. This system is different from the other genome editing tools such as ZFNs and TALENs, and thus synthesis of sgRNA is a *prerequisite* for this system. This development dramatically reduced both the complexity and time required for the design and implementation of gene editing.

3. History of GE in pigs

Table 1 lists instances of production of GE piglets with genome editing technology from 2011 to 2018. This section provides a brief explanation on the background of GE pig production.

In 2011, three types of GE piglets were produced using ZFNs from different laboratories. All of these piglets were produced by SCNT using GE cells as a SCNT donor. The first report showing successful production of GE piglets involved the disruption of enhanced green fluorescent protein (*EGFP*) gene in a hemizygous manner. Whyte et al. [41] demonstrated that a ZFN pair efficiently inactivated the expression of *EGFP* that was integrated into the chromosomes of porcine fibroblasts via the NHEJ pathway with an efficiency of ~5%. From this experiment, it

Method	Genome editing tool (mode for gene modification)	Method for gene modification	Outcome	Target gene	References
SCNT	ZFN (indels)	Using adult porcine ear fibroblasts hemizygous for the eGFP transgene	Seven of nine embryos (Day 12) exhibited loss of fluorescence	*eGFP* transgene	[41]
SCNT	ZFN (indels)	Using porcine fibroblasts transfected with ZFN plasmid	Of 10 live piglets delivered, two carried the predicted ZFN-induced mutation; lower expression of both *PPAR-γ1* and *PPAR-γ2* was observed in those clones	*PPARγ*	[42]
SCNT	ZFN (indels)	Using porcine fetal fibroblasts transfected with ZFN plasmid	Of six fetuses, all completely lacked α-Gal epitopes	*GGTA1*	[43]
MI	TALEN (indels)	Cytoplasmic MI of TALEN mRNA toward IVF-derived zygotes	CI of TALEN mRNAs inducing gene KO in up to 75% of embryos; Of the 18 live-born clones, eight contained monoallelic mutations and 10 contained biallelic modifications of the *LDLR* gene	*LDLR*	[44]
MI	ZFN, TALEN (indels)	Cytoplasmic MI of ZFN or TALEN mRNA toward *in vivo* fertilized zygotes	Of 39 piglets produced, eight carried TALEN-derived editing events (21%); of nine piglets produced, one carried an editing event at the ZFN target site (11%)	*NF-kappaB subunit*	[45]
SCNT	TALENs (indels)	Using porcine fetal fibroblasts transfected with TALEN plasmid	Three piglets with biallelic mutations of the *GGTA1* gene exhibited loss of α-Gal epitopes on the surface of cells	*GGTA1*	[46]
SCNT	TALENs (indels/KI)	Using porcine fibroblasts transfected with TALEN mRNA + ssODN	Of eight piglets born from *DAZL*-modified cells, three are still born; of the six piglets from *APC*-modified cells, only one alive	*DAZL*, *APC*	[47]
SCNT	ZFNs (indels)	Using porcine fetal fibroblasts transfected with ZFN mRNA	The resulting *IL2RG* KO pigs completely lacked a thymus and were deficient in T and NK cells, similar to human X-linked SCID patients	*IL2RG*	[48]
SCNT	ZFN (indels)	Using porcine adult liver-derived cells transfected with ZFN plasmid through the two-steps	Four viable and healthy cloned pigs obtained exhibited disruption of the *GGTA1* and the *CMAH* loci	*GGTA1*, *CMAH*	[49]
SCNT	ZFN (KI)	Using porcine fibroblast cells transfected with ZFN plasmid and donor DNA	Successfully produced healthy monoallelic/biallelic CMAH KO pigs	*CMAH*	[50]

Method	Genome editing tool (mode for gene modification)	Method for gene modification	Outcome	Target gene	References
SCNT/MI	CRISPR/Cas9 (KI/indels)	Using porcine fetal fibroblasts transfected with sgRNA-Cas9 plasmids + donor DNA/cytoplasmic MI of Cas9 mRNA/sgRNA toward IVF-derived zygotes	Of the *CD163* recipients, five delivered healthy piglets by cesarean section; 12 of the 13 piglets contained either a biallelic or homozygous deletion of *CD1D*	*eGFP*, *CD163*, *CD1D*	[51]
MI	CRISPR/Cas9 (indels)	Cytoplasmic MI of Cas9 mRNA/sgRNA toward *in vivo* fertilized zygotes	Ten of 16 resulting piglets had indels with an efficiency of 63% and were comprised by cells with monoallelic mutant; they can be a model for von Willebrand disease	*vWF*	[52]
SCNT	CRISPR/Cas9 (indels)	Using porcine fetal fibroblasts transfected with Cas9/sgRNA expression plasmid	A total of three piglets were obtained; fibroblasts from all three animals were negative for class I SLA cell surface expression	*class I MHC*	[53]
SCNT	TALENs (indels)	Using pig fetal fibroblasts transfected with TALEN plasmid	Of 27 live cloned piglets obtained, nine were targeted with biallelic mutations in *RAG1*, three were targeted with biallelic mutations in *RAG2*, and 10 were targeted with a monoallelic mutation in *RAG2*	*RAG1*, *RAG2*	[54]
SCNT	ZFN (indels)	Using pig fetal fibroblasts transfected with ZFN plasmid	Three *GGTA1* null piglets showing loss of α-Gal epitope expression were born	*GGTA1*	[55]
SCNT	CRISPR/Cas9 (indels)	Using pig liver-derived cells transfected with two or three plasmids expressing Cas9 and sgRNA targeting to GGTA1, CMAH, or putative iGb3S genes	Of 10 fetuses obtained, five had mutations in both the *GGTA1* and *CMAH* genes	*GGTA1*, *CMAH*, *putative iGb3S*	[56]
SCNT	ZFNs (indels)	Using pig fetal fibroblasts transfected with ZFN plasmid	The *MSTN*-mutant pigs grew normally, had increased muscle mass with decreased fat accumulation	*MSTN*	[57]
SCNT	TALENs (indels)	Using pig liver-derived cells transfected with TALEN plasmid	Livers from *ASGR1*−/− pigs exhibit decreased human platelet uptake	*ASGR1*	[58]
SCNT	ZFN/TALEN (indels)	Using pig fetal fibroblasts transfected with TALEN or ZFN mRNA	One of the cloned pigs generated GalT/CMAH-double homozygous KO pigs	*CMAH*	[59]
SCNT	CRISPR/Cas9 (KI)	Using pig fetal fibroblasts transfected with targeting donor vector and two expression vectors for sgRNA and Cas9	Highly efficient KI (up to 54%) was achieved after drug selection; one cloned piglet obtained showed correct targeting	*H11*	[60]

Method	Genome editing tool (mode for gene modification)	Method for gene modification	Outcome	Target gene	References
SCNT	CRISPR/Cas9	Using pig fetal fibroblasts transfected with sgRNA, Cas9 expression plasmids	Four cloned double KO piglets showing loss of expression for both *PARK2* and *PINK1* were produced	*TYR*, *PARK2*, *PINK1*	[61]
MI	CRISPR/Cas9 (KI)	Cytoplasmic MI of Cas9 mRNA + sgRNA + ssODN toward *in vivo* fertilized zygotes	Two live-born piglets obtained showed the white coat-color phenotype over its entire body	*MITF*	[62]
MI	CRISPR/Cas9 (KI)	Cytoplasmic MI of Cas9 mRNA + sgRNA + circular vector toward *in vivo* fertilized zygotes	All 16 piglets born were healthy and carried the expected KI allele; the KI allele was successfully transmitted through germline	*Alb*	[63]
MI	CRISPR/Cas9 (indels)	Cytoplasmic MI of Cas9 mRNA and sgRNA toward *in vivo* fertilized zygotes	Bi-allelic modifications of pig *Npc1l1* were achieved at the efficiency as high as 100%	*Npc1l1*	[64]
SCNT	CRISPR/Cas9 (indels)	Using pig fetal fibroblasts transfected with sgRNA-Cas9 encoding vector	Of eight marker-gene-free cloned pigs with biallelic mutations obtained, some showed phenotypes similar to DM	*MSTN*	[65]
SCNT	CRISPR/Cas9 (indels)	Using liver-derived cells transfected with sgRNA-Cas9 encoding vectors	One triple knockout pig was obtained; Cells from this cloned pig exhibited reduced human IgM and IgG binding	*GGTA1*, *CMAH*, *β4GalNT2*	[66]
SCNT	CRISPR/Cas9 (indels)	Using pig fetal fibroblasts transfected with sgRNA-Cas9 encoding vector	Three cloned piglets with biallelic mutation produced showed no antibody-producing B cells	*IgM* J_H	[67]
EP	CRISPR/Cas9 (indels)	Using Cas9 protein and sgRNA (RNP) toward IVF-derived zygotes	The use of gene editing by electroporation of Cas9 protein (GEEP) resulted in highly efficient targeted gene disruption and efficient production of *Myostatin* mutant pigs	*MSTN*	[68]
MI	CRISPR/Cas9 (indels)	Cytoplasmic MI of Cas9 mRNA and sgRNA toward *in vivo* fertilized zygotes	Of two piglets obtained, one piglets exhibited *DMD* phenotype, as exemplified by degenerative and disordered skeletal and cardiac muscle	*DMD*	[69]
SCNT	ZFN (indels)	Using pig fetal fibroblasts transfected with ZFN-encoding mRNA	The heterozygous *FBN1* mutant pigs obtained exhibited abnormal phenotype, which resembles MFS found in humans	*FBN1*	[70]

Method	Genome editing tool (mode for gene modification)	Method for gene modification	Outcome	Target gene	References
SCNT	CRISPR/Cas9 (KI)	Using pig fetal fibroblasts transfected with Cas9-sgRNA expression vector + donor DNA containing Cre/loxP system	Two male live piglets with mono-allelic *MSTN* KO obtained exhibited enhanced myofiber quantity, but the myofiber size remained unaltered	*MSTN*	[71]
SCNT	TALENs (indels)	Using pig fetal fibroblasts transfected with TALEN plasmids	In total, 12 live and two stillborn piglets were collected; all fetuses and piglets exhibited homozygous *GGTA1*-null mutation	*GGTA1*	[72]
SCNT	TALENs (indels)	Using porcine fetal fibroblasts co-transfected with TALEN and hDAF expression plasmids	Six live-born piglets and three stillborn piglets were obtained; the piglets showed eight base mono-allelic mutations of *GGTA1* and *hDAF* expression	*GGTA1*	[73]
SCNT	CRISPR/Cas9 (indels)	Using fetal fibroblast cells transfected with sgRNA-Cas9 encoding vector	Four live *RUNX3* KO piglets with monoallelic mutation showed the lack of RUNX3 protein in their internal organ system	*RUNX3*	[74]
SCNT	TALENs (indels)	Using dermal fibroblasts transfected with TALEN plasmids	*MSTN* KO piglets exhibited a double-muscled phenotype, possessing a higher body weight and longissimus muscle mass measuring 170% that of wild-type piglets, with double the number of muscle fibers	*MSTN*	[75]
SCNT	TALENs/Cas9 (KI)	Using fetal fibroblast cells transfected with Cas9/sgRNA or TALEN vector + ssODN	Of seven cloned piglets, some expressed human insulin	*INS*	[76]
SCNT	CRISPR/Cas9 (KI)	Using fetal fibroblast cells transfected with sgRNA-Cas9 encoding vector + ssODN	One cloned stillborn piglet harbored the orthologous p.C313Y mutation at the *MSTN* locus	*APP*, *LRRK2*, MSTN	[77]
SCNT	TALENs (indels)	Using ear fibroblasts transfected with TALEN vectors	Thirty *GGTA1* biallelic KO piglets were successfully delivered and grew normally.	*GGTA1*	[78]
MI	CRISPR/Cas9 (KI)	Cytoplasmic MI of Cas9 mRNA + sgRNA + ssODN toward *in vivo* fertilized zygotes	Of five piglets delivered alive, three exhibited pigmentary disorders with light-colored iris in eye, which was observed in patients harboring *Sox10* mutations	*Sox10*	[79]
MI	CRISPR/Cas9 (indels)	Cytoplasmic MI of sgRNA-Cas9 encoding vector toward *in vivo* fertilized zygotes	Of six healthy fetuses recovered, four exhibited loss of α-Gal epitope expression, indicating a biallelic KO of *GGTA1*	*GGTA1*	[80]

Method	Genome editing tool (mode for gene modification)	Method for gene modification	Outcome	Target gene	References
MI	CRISPR/Cas9 (indels)	Cytoplasmic MI of Cas9 mRNA + three types of sgRNAs toward *in vivo* fertilized zygotes	Of two live-born piglets delivered, one piglet showed biallelic modification of all three genes, and another showed biallelic modification of the *DJ-1* and *PINK1* genes and monoallelic mutations of *parkin* gene	*Parkin*, *DJ-1*, *PINK1*	[81]
SCNT-MI	CRISPR/Cas9 (indels)	Cytoplasmic MI of RNP toward SCNT embryos	Six fetuses recovered revealed that all fetuses carried biallelic edits for the *GRB10* gene (6/6, 100%)	*GRB10*	[82]
SCNT	CRISPR/Cas9 (indels)	Using kidney fibroblasts transfected with ZFN vectors	Two healthy normal females with *GGTA1*, *CMAH* double KO phenotypes are currently being raised for mating	*GGTA1*, *CMAH*	[83]
MI	CRISPR/Cas9 (indels)	Cytoplasmic MI of Cas9 mRNA + sgRNA toward IVF-derived zygotes	Seventeen live piglets and two stillborn were produced; all had mutations in both genes (no pigs with wild-type sequence)	*RAG2*, *IL2RG*	[84]
MI	CRISPR/Cas9 (indels)	Cytoplasmic MI of Cas9 mRNA + sgRNA toward *in vivo* fertilized zygotes	Eighteen piglets recovered showed either mono- or bi-allelic modifications and no wild-type animals; *NANOS2* KO pigs phenocopied KO mice with male specific germline ablation	*NANOS2*	[85]
SCNT	CRISPR/Cas9 (indels)	Using fetal fibroblasts transfected with sgRNA and Cas9 expression vectors	Six biallelic KO pigs with mutations in *ApoE* and *LDLR* genes were obtained successfully in a single step.	*ApoE*, *LDLR*	[86]
SCNT	TALENs	Using fetal fibroblasts transfected with TALEN plasmid	All six live piglets obtained carried biallelic mutations in the *P53* locus	*P53*	[87]
SCNT	TALEN (indels)	Using fetal fibroblasts transfected with TALEN plasmid	A total of 18 live piglets were obtained; they showed hypermuscular characteristics	*MSTN*	[88]
SCNT	CRISPR/Cas9 (indels)	Using fetal fibroblasts transfected with sgRNA-Cas9 encoding vectors	A total of 37 PERV-inactivated piglets were generated; 15 piglets remain alive	*PERV*	[89]

Method	Genome editing tool (mode for gene modification)	Method for gene modification	Outcome	Target gene	References
SCNT	CRISPR/Cas9 (indels)	Using fetal fibroblasts transfected with sgRNA-Cas9 encoding vectors	Of 26 female piglets delivered, 23 piglets carried mutations in the *MSTN* locus; the bi-allelic KO pigs were viable and exhibited partial double-muscled phenotype	*MSTN*	[90]
SCNT	CRISPR/Cas9 (KI)	Using fetal fibroblasts transfected with Cas9-gRNA plasmid and targeting vector	Twelve male piglets were born and expressed *UCP1* in a tissue-specific manner	*UCP1*	[91]
MI	CRISPR/Cas9 (KI)	Cytoplasmic MI of RNP toward *in vivo* fertilized zygotes	A total of 18 fetuses/born piglets were obtained; successful insertion of pseudo *attP* sites within the *COL1A* locus was observed	*COL1A*	[92]
MI	CRISPR/Cas9 (indels)	Cytoplasmic MI of Cas9 mRNA + sgRNAs toward *in vivo*-derived zygotes	Indels in 92–100% of the embryos analyzed; all resulting 12 piglets had biallelic edits of *TMRPSS2*	*TMPRSS2*	[93]
MI	CRISPR/Cas9 (indels)	Direct pronuclear microinjection of Cas9-gRNA plasmid	Of seven born piglets, one exhibited biallelic KO phenotype and one did monoallelic KO one	*GGTA1*	[94]
MI	CRISPR/Cas9 (indels)	Cytoplasmic MI of Cas9 mRNA and dual sgRNAs toward *in vivo* fertilized zygotes	Of nine fetuses examined, three exhibited bi-allelic mutations at the *PDX1* locus; in those fetuses pancreatic primordium was highly disorganized	*PDX1*	[95]
SCNT (Handmade cloning)	CRISPR/Cas9 (indels)	Using fetal fibroblasts transfected with sgRNA and Cas9 expression vectors	Eleven live bi-allelic *GGTA1/CMAH* double KO piglets were obtained with the identical phenotype	*GGTA1*, *CMAH*	[96]
EP	CRISPR/Cas9	Using Cas9 protein and sgRNA (RNP) toward IVF-derived zygotes	Of 11 piglets born, nine survived; six of nine carried mutations in *TP53*; three of the genome-edited pigs (50%) exhibited various tumor phenotypes	*TP53*	[97]
SCNT	CRISPR/Cas9 (KI)	Using fetal fibroblasts transfected with sgRNA- Cas9 plasmid + donor DNA	Three piglets born grew and developed normally; all these piglets had *fat-1* KI at the Rosa26 locus	*Rosa26*	[98]
SCNT	CRISPR/Cas9 (KI)	Using fetal fibroblasts transfected with sgRNA- Cas9 plasmid + donor DNA	Of seven naturally delivered piglets, six showed successful KI; the KI allele was successfully transmitted through germline	*HTT*	[99]

Method	Genome editing tool (mode for gene modification)	Method for gene modification	Outcome	Target gene	References
SCNT	CRISPR/Cas9 (indels)	Using fetal fibroblasts transfected with sgRNA- Cas9 plasmid	Of a total of 17 piglets obtained, 12 appeared healthy; all had mutations at the target locus	*FBXO40*	[100]

Abbreviations: APC, adenomatous polyposis coli; Alb, albumin; GGTA1, α-1,3-galactosyltransferase gene; APP, amyloid precursor protein; ApoE, apolipoprotein E; ASGR1, asialoglycoprotein receptor; β4GalNT2, β1,4-N-acetylgalactosaminyl transferase; class I MHC, class I major histocompatibility complex; CRISPR/Cas9, clustered regulated interspaced short palindromic repeat and CRISPR-associated Cas; COL1A, collagen type I alpha 1 chain; CMAH, cytidine monophosphate-N-acetylneuraminic acid hydroxylase; DAZL, deleted in azoospermia-like; DM, double muscling; DMD, Duchenne muscular dystrophy; PARKIN, E3 ubiquitin ligase PARK2; EP, electroporation; eGFP, enhanced green fluorescent protein; FBXO40, F-box protein 40; FBN1, fibrillin-1; GM, gene-modified; GRB10, growth-hormone receptor binding protein-10; H11, Hipp11; hDAF, human decay-accelerating factor; HTT, huntingtin; indels, insertion or deletion of nucleotides; INS, insulin; IL2RG, interleukin-2 receptor gamma; IVF, in vitro fertilized; iGb3S, isogloboside 3 synthase; IgM J_H, JH region of the pig IgM heavy chain; KI, knock-in; KO, knockout; LRRK2, leucine-rich repeat kinase 2; LDLR, low density lipoprotein receptor; MFS, Marfan syndrome; MI, microinjection; SCNT-MI, microinjection following somatic cell nuclear transfer; MITF, Microphthalmia-associated transcription factor; MSTN, myostatin; NANOS2, nanos C2HC-type zinc finger 2; fat-1, n-3 fatty acid desaturase; Npc1l1, Niemann-Pick C1-Like 1; PDX-1, pancreas duodenum homeobox 1; DJ-1, PARK7; PARK2, parkin; PPARγ, peroxisome proliferator-activated receptor-gamma; PERV, porcine endogenous retrovirus; PINK1, PTEN-induced putative kinase 1; RNP, ribonucleoprotein; RUNX3, Runt-related transcription factor 3; sgRNA, single guide RNA; ssODN, single-stranded DNA oligonucleotides; SCNT, somatic cell nuclear transfer; Sox10, SRY (sex determining region Y)-box 10; TALENs, transcription activator-like effector nucleases; TMPRSS2, transmembrane protease, serine S1, member 2; TYR, tyrosinase; UCP1, uncoupling protein 1; vWF, von Willebrand factor; ZFNs, zinc finger nucleases.

Table 1.
Summary of production of genome-edited pigs.

was found that the endogenous NHEJ pathway is effective for inducing mutation in a porcine target gene. Furthermore, SCNT using GE cells with the mutated allele as a SCNT donor demonstrated that seven of the nine resulting cloned fetuses (at Day 12) stopped expressing EGFP. Yang et al. [42] co-transfected porcine fibroblasts with ZFN and pcDNA3.1 plasmids (providing *neo*) by electroporation (EP), performed SCNT using these GE cells, and finally obtained peroxisome proliferator-activated receptor γ (PPARγ) mono-allelic KO pigs, which are expected to generate a porcine cardiomyopathy model. Hauschild et al. [43] attempted to destroy *GGTA1*, an endogenous gene encoding an enzyme required for production of a xenogeneic antigen called α-Gal epitope, using ZFNs in porcine fetal cells. They found that α-Gal epitope-negative cells with the bi-allelic KO phenotype can be efficiently isolated by FACS, and the resultant GE cells have the potential to make cloned piglets. Importantly, this experiment suggests that it is possible to produce individuals with a bi-allelic KO phenotype with this technology. In other words, bi-allelic KO piglets can be directly created without breeding or subcloning, which contrasts with past instances where only heterozygous KO piglets have been produced through traditional gene targeting. Hauschild et al. [43] also showed that neither off-target cleavage nor integration of the ZFN-coding plasmid occurred.

The successful production of genome-edited piglets with bi-allelic KO genotype obtained after cytoplasmic MI of *in vivo*-derived porcine zygotes using either ZFN or TALEN mRNA was first reported by Lillico et al. [45]. This MI-based production of GE animals was also shown to be successful in mice [101–104].

Hai et al. [52] first demonstrated that GE pigs can be produced using the CRISPR/Cas9 system. They performed cytoplasmic MI with Cas9 mRNA and sgRNA targeted to *von Willebrand factor* gene (*vWF*) to produce a pig *model* for type 1 von Willebrand disease. In this study, 10 of 16 resulting piglets had indels with an efficiency of 63%, and most pigs contained more than two different alleles, suggesting mono-allelic mutants.

Successful knock-in (KI) of a GOI into the target locus was first reported in pigs by Ruan et al. [60] and Peng et al. [63]. Zhou et al. [61] demonstrated the production of SCNT-treated piglets with mutations in multiple genes after a single transfection.

Fischer et al. [83] first succeeded in producing GE pigs by cytoplasmic MI of a Cas9 protein/gRNA complex called a ribonucleoprotein (RNP). Furthermore, GE pigs could be efficiently produced by *in vitro* EP in the presence of RNP [68]. Sheets et al. [82] produced GE fetuses by cytoplasmic MI of RNP into oocytes reconstituted with intact cells using the SCNT technology. By this treatment, they reported highly efficient (100%) generation of bi-allelic modification in the resultant cloned fetuses. The significance of this approach is be that researchers can obtain GE pigs with a defined genetic background, even though the starting oocytes are derived from ovaries obtained from a slaughterhouse.

4. Delivery method

For the production of GE pigs, the choice of delivery method for genome editing components in porcine zygotes is important. As shown in **Table 1**, the methods for the production of GE pigs achieved by delivering genome editing reagents at earlier stages of development can be largely divided into four groups: the first is MI of genome editing reagents (in a form of DNA, mRNA or protein) into zygotes (**Figure 1A**); the second is SCNT using GE cells as the SCNT donor (**Figure 1B**); the third is *in vitro* EP of zygotes in the presence of genome editing reagents (**Figure 1C**); the fourth is MI of genome editing reagents into SCNT-treated

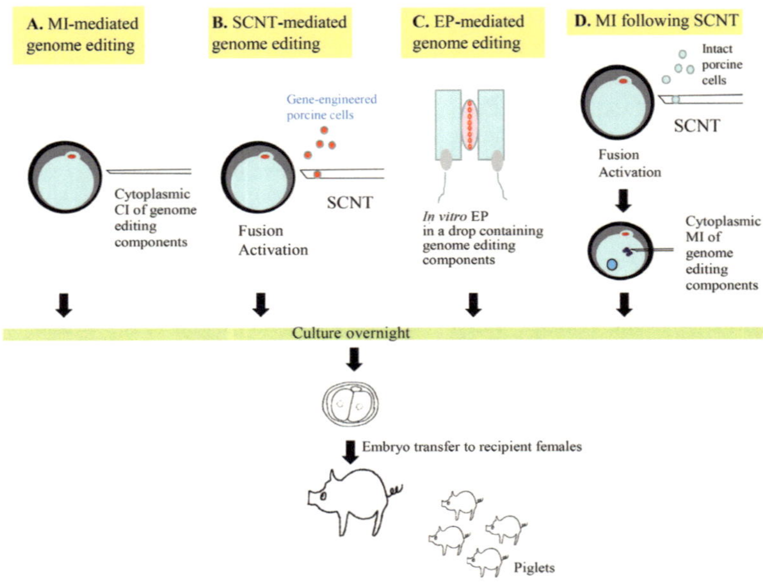

Figure 1.
Several methods to create genome-edited pigs. (A) Microinjection (MI)-based method using zygotes. (B) Somatic cell nuclear transfer (SCNT)-based method using gene-engineered (GE) cells as a SCNT donor. (C) Electroporation (EP)-based method using zygotes. (D) MI-based method using the SCNT-treated embryos.

embryos reconstituted using a normal cell (**Figure 1D**). Furthermore, we will provide a new approach based on *in vitro* EP of the SCNT-treated embryos reconstituted using a normal cell as the fifth group of methods for possible production of GE pigs (**Figure 2A**). In the following sections, each of these methods are described.

4.1 MI

MI is an important tool in the creation of GE piglets. To date, about 30% (17/60) of studies (**Table 1**) have employed this approach. For example, in the case of MI with CRISPR/Cas9-related mRNA, a single cytoplasmic MI of 2–10 pL containing 125 ng/μL Cas9 mRNA and 12.5 ng/μL sgRNA was adopted [62]. Yu et al. [69] employed Cas9 mRNA (20 ng/μL) and sgRNA (10 ng/μL) mixtures for cytoplasmic MI.

Is MI of these components deleterious to the development of porcine zygotes? According to Hai et al. [52], the *in vitro* developmental efficiencies of embryos injected with Cas9 mRNA/sgRNA (~79%) and embryos injected with water (~77%) were both very high and comparable with each other, suggesting that the MI and the Cas9 mRNA/sgRNA had little effect on early embryonic development. On the contrary, Whitworth et al. [51] reported that a higher concentration of sgRNA induces toxicity in porcine embryos. According to Whitworth et al. [51], 10 ng/μL of sgRNA and Cas9 mRNA are recommended.

Selecting appropriate zygotes also appears to be an important factor in the production of GE pigs. For acquisition of viable zygotes, there are at least two methods. One is isolation of zygotes from oviducts of a female that has been inseminated, hereinafter called "*in vivo*-derived zygotes," and the other is acquisition of zygotes by *in vitro* fertilization (IVF) between *in vitro* matured oocytes (derived from the ovaries obtained from the slaughterhouse) and sperm. Generally, it is believed that the *in vivo*-derived zygotes exhibit superior development performance comparing to the IVF-derived zygotes [51, 62]. Indeed, the number of laboratories using

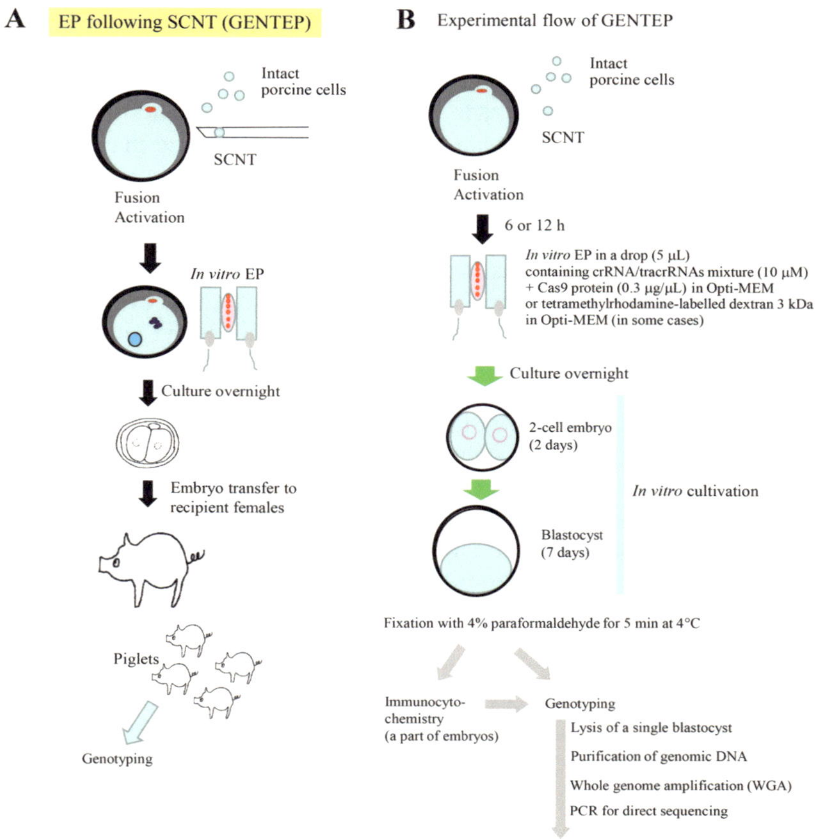

Figure 2.
A new method for production of genome-edited pigs. (A) EP-based method using the SCNT-treated embryos, which is termed "GENTEP." (B) Experimental outline for checking the validity of GENTEP.

IVF-derived zygotes for production of GE pigs is low (~30% (5/17); see **Table 1**). However, acquisition of viable *in vivo*-derived zygotes is laborious and often associated with the sacrifice of pregnant females, which appears to be one of the major goals for improvement in genetic engineering technology using pigs.

The frequent generation of individuals with mosaic genotypes is also a serious problem associated with MI-based GE pig production. Sato et al. [105] demonstrated that cytoplasmic MI of parthenogenetically activated porcine embryos (hereinafter called "parthenotes") with Cas9 mRNA + sgRNA caused frequent mosaicism in the offspring (blastocysts) with cells with mixed genotype, so-called normal wild-type cells and mutated cells, when they were subjected to cytoplasmic MI immediately after oocyte activation. Notably, Carlson et al. [44] suggested that 100% of bovine embryos exhibited fluorescence expression after cytoplasmic MI of *EGFP* mRNA, but only ~40% of porcine embryos did. It is probable that an endogenous system for translation to protein from mRNA may not be sufficiently established in those porcine embryos, especially at the stage immediately after fertilization or zygotic activation. Indeed, Sato et al. [106] demonstrated that this mosaicism can be partially improved when cytoplasmic MI is performed with oocytes 12 h after activation. In contrast, other researchers reported that only 10–20% of MI-treated embryos exhibited mosaicism [51, 84]. Notably, Whitworth et al. [51] performed cytoplasmic MI with Cas9 mRNA + sgRNA toward fertilized oocytes at 14 h post-fertilization. In this context, the use of sgRNA and an RNP instead of Cas9 mRNA may be the key to solving this issue of mosaicism, as the Cas9 protein is more rapidly translated, folded, and complexed with sgRNAs prior to editing, unlike the Cas9 mRNA [107–109]. For example, in mice, delivering RNPs into zygotes causes rapid genome editing in the target locus, which also maximizes efficiency while minimizing mosaicism [110–112]. Indeed, Sheets et al. [82] demonstrated that after MI with RNP, 100% of piglets produced had the bi-allelic KO genotype.

Interestingly, Petersen et al. [80] demonstrated that cytoplasmic MI of DNA vectors coding for CRISPR/Cas9 targeting the porcine *GGTA1* gene enabled biallelic knockout of *GGTA1* in 7/12 fetuses and piglets (58.3%). As mentioned previously, it is difficult to visualize porcine pronuclei at zygote stage under normal conditions due to high lipid content in the cytoplasm. Researchers therefore must centrifuge them briefly prior to MI. The fact that cytoplasmic MI of DNA vectors can induce genome editing at a target locus may be beneficial for researchers, because preparation of plasmid DNA is easier than that of mRNA, and it is generally more resistant against degradation than mRNA. According to Petersen et al. [80], it currently remains unknown how the circular DNA plasmid translocates from the cytoplasm to the nucleus. They speculate that the SV40 nuclear translocation signal of the CRISPR/Cas9 plasmid could play an important role by facilitating nuclear translocation via association with ubiquitous transcription factors.

4.2 SCNT

SCNT using GE cells as an SCNT donor is another way to produce GE pigs. The merit of this approach is the use of *in vitro* cultivated cells such as fetal fibroblasts to which various genetic engineering techniques (i.e., introduction of multiple KO, KI, and transgenes) can be applied easily. After gene transfer, these cells are subjected to cell selection through drug selection or fluorescence activated cell sorting (FACS) to enrich GE cells as a pure population. Thus, it is highly probable that the resulting SCNT-derived GE founder pigs have a predictable genotype and low rates of mosaicism. Unfortunately, as mentioned previously, the efficiency of SCNT to produce cloned piglets is still very low. Much effort has been focused on improving the low efficiency associated with the SCNT, which includes improvement of the oocyte/zygote culture system and application of chemical reagents to alter the epigenetic status of transferred nuclei. For improving the culture method, researchers have used vitamin C [113], α-tocopherol [114], melatonin [115] or alanyl-glutamine dipeptide (instead of glutamine) [116]. For altering the epigenetic status, researchers have used histone deacetylase inhibitors (HDACi) such as trichostatin A (TSA) [117, 118], valproic acid (VPA) [119–121], scriptaid [122–124], LBH589 (panobinostat) [125], oxamflatin [126], PXD101 (belinostat) [127], quisinostat [128], MGCD0103 [129], or histone methyltransferase inhibitors such as MM-102 [130]. Lin et al. [131] employed tauroursodeoxycholic acid (TUDCA), an inhibitor of endoplasmic reticulum (ER) stress, and demonstrated that TUDCA can enhance the developmental potential of porcine SCNT embryos by attenuating ER stress and reducing apoptosis. Wang et al. [132] demonstrated that administration of siRNA or microRNA-148a, both of which can suppress the function of DNA methyltransferase 1 (*DNMT1*) at a transcriptional level, is effective for enhancing the developmental potential of SCNT embryos. Furthermore, Matoba et al. [133] succeeded in drastically increasing SCNT efficiency by cytoplasmic MI of mRNA coding for histone demethylase (*Kdm4d*) in mice.

4.3 EP

EP is known to be a useful and powerful gene delivery tool enabling transfer of exogenous substances (i.e., DNA) into a cell and was first applied to rat zygotes for genome editing by Kaneko et al. [134]. Since then, many researchers have successfully induced gene edits by using this technology in mice [135, 136], bovines [137] and pigs [68]. The merit of this technology is that it is simple, rapid and convenient for genome editing in zygotes, compared to the previous MI-based technique. Notably, about 30–50 zygotes can be edited with one pulse of EP. Furthermore, EP only requires a square pulse generator called an electroporator, and not a more expensive micromanipulator system.

As mentioned previously, Tanihara et al. [68] first applied EP to porcine IVF-derived zygotes and produced genome-edited pigs. They used CRISPR/Cas9-based RNP for knock-in of a target gene, and achieved reduced mosaicism and higher efficiency of genome-edited pig production with EP (30 V, square pulse 1.0 ms in duration repeated five times) using an electrode (#LF501PT1-20; BEX Co. Ltd., Tokyo, Japan) connected to a CUY21EDIT II electroporator (BEX Co. Ltd.). Notably, they reported no appreciable reduction in the developmental ability of the EP-treated embryos.

4.4 MI after SCNT

Although direct modification of zygotic genomes provides some advantages, SCNT also provides a significant advantage by permitting the isolation of cells containing precise modifications before the expense of animal production is incurred. As mentioned previously, Sheets et al. [82] successfully produced genome-edited cloned pigs by combining SCNT with CRISPR/Cas9 MI, which is beneficial for researchers as they do not need to manage a founder herd, and can eliminate the need for laborious *in vitro* culture and screening. In this study, all (6/6) of the resultant clone fetuses exhibited 100% bi-allelic modification. Unfortunately, they failed to describe successful production of *live birth piglets*, but it seems that this approach is a powerful tool for GE pig production.

4.5 EP after SCNT

Similar to the approach shown by Sheets et al. [82], we tried to obtain cloned GE piglets through *in vitro* EP in the SCNT-treated embryos, which is called Genome Editing via Nuclear Transfer and subsequent Electroporation or GENTEP (**Figure 2A**). Some results obtained from GENTEP-related experiments are presented below.

SCNT-derived embryos were obtained by inserting fetal fibroblasts derived from microminiature pigs (MMP) [138] into the perivitelline space between enucleated porcine oocytes (derived from ovaries obtained from a slaughterhouse) and zona pellucida, according to the method described by Miyoshi et al. [119] (**Figure 2B**). The resulting SCNT-derived embryos were then subjected to electric activation following electric fusion between an egg and a cell (**Figure 2B**). Six or 12 h after activation, the SCNT-treated embryos were subjected to *in vitro* EP in the presence of RNP targeted to the pig low density lipoprotein receptor (*LDLR*) gene (**Figure 2B**). Parthenotes (~6 h after electric activation) were also used for *in vitro* EP using tetramethylrhodamine-labeled dextran 3 kDa (used as an indicator for successful gene delivery) (as shown in **Figure 3A**) or as controls for immunocytochemistry using anti-LDLR antibody (as shown in **Figure 3B**).

First, we examined whether the *in vitro* EP we used here is effective for successful gene delivery to porcine embryos and does not cause any deleterious effects on their embryonic development, using porcine parthenotes (6 h after activation). The EP procedure was based on the method described by Hashimoto and Takemoto [135]. An electroporation chamber (#LF610P4-4_470; BEX Co. Ltd.), in which two platinum block electrodes were situated with a 1-mm gap between them (**Figure 1C**), was placed under a stereoscopic microscope and connected to

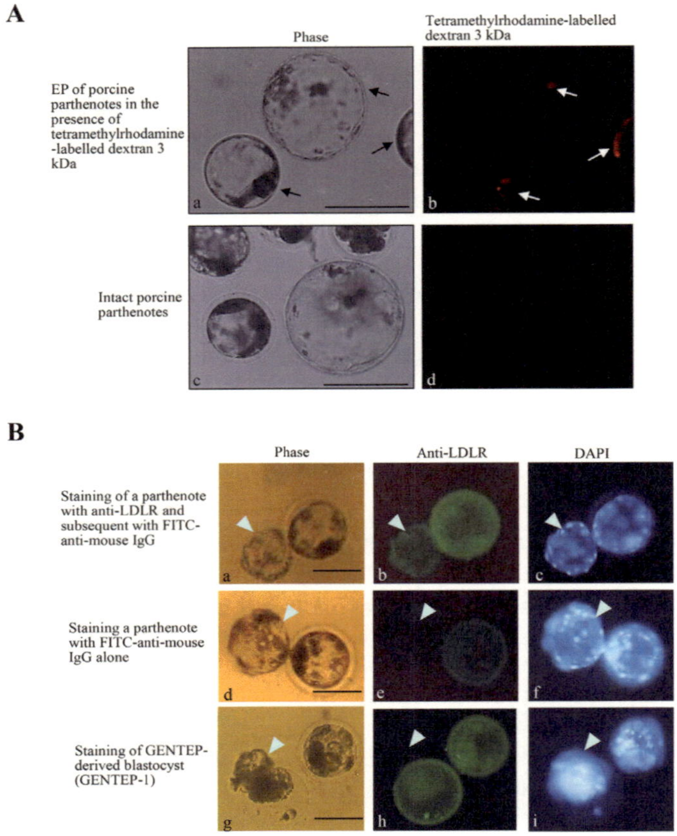

Figure 3.
Validity check of GENTEP. (A) EP of parthenotes (6 h after activation) in the presence of tetramethylrhodamine-labelled dextran 3 kDa. Porcine parthenotes were subjected to in vitro *EP, and then cultured for 7 days up to blastocysts. Note that almost all of the EP-treated blastocysts are fluorescent (arrows in a and b), while intact parthenotes do not fluoresce (c and d). Bar = 100 μm. (B) Staining with anti-LDLR antibody. The intact parthenote (hatched blastocysts) exhibits the reactivity to the antibody (arrowheads in a–c), but not to the second antibody alone (arrowheads in d–f). No reactivity to the antibody was also seen in the GENTEP-derived blastocyst (arrowheads in g–i). Nuclear staining with DAPI was performed after staining with the second antibody. Note that porcine zona pellucida was slightly stained with the second antibody, since it was found to be reactive with the second antibody alone (see d–f). Bar = 100 μm.*

an electric pulse generator (CUY21EDITII Genome Editor™, BEX Co. Ltd.). About 20 parthenotes were placed into a 5-μL drop containing 2 μg/μL tetramethylrhodamine-dextran 3 kDa (#D3307; Thermo Fisher Scientific Inc., Waltham, MA, USA) in Opti-MEM (Invitrogen, Carlsbad, CA, USA) between the electrodes (**Figure 1C**). EP was performed under these conditions: 30 V, square pulses, 1.0 ms in duration at 99 ms intervals, repeated seven times. The EP-treated parthenotes were then cultured for 7 days up to blastocysts to evaluate the *in vitro* developmental rate and uptake of fluorescent dye into the embryos. Approximately 40% of the EP-treated parthenotes developed to the blastocyst stage and ~80% of them exhibited bright tetramethylrhodamine-derived fluorescence [arrows in **Figure 3A(a,b)**]. This result suggests that our EP condition is useful for effective delivery of a foreign substance into porcine embryos and not harmful for their development.

Second, we performed CRISPR/Cas9-based genome editing (targeted to the endogenous *LDLR* gene) with porcine SCNT-treated embryos. We designed sgRNA capable of recognizing a 20 bp sequence spanning the translation initiation codon (ATG) upstream of the protospacer adjacent motif (PAM) sequence (CGG) on the

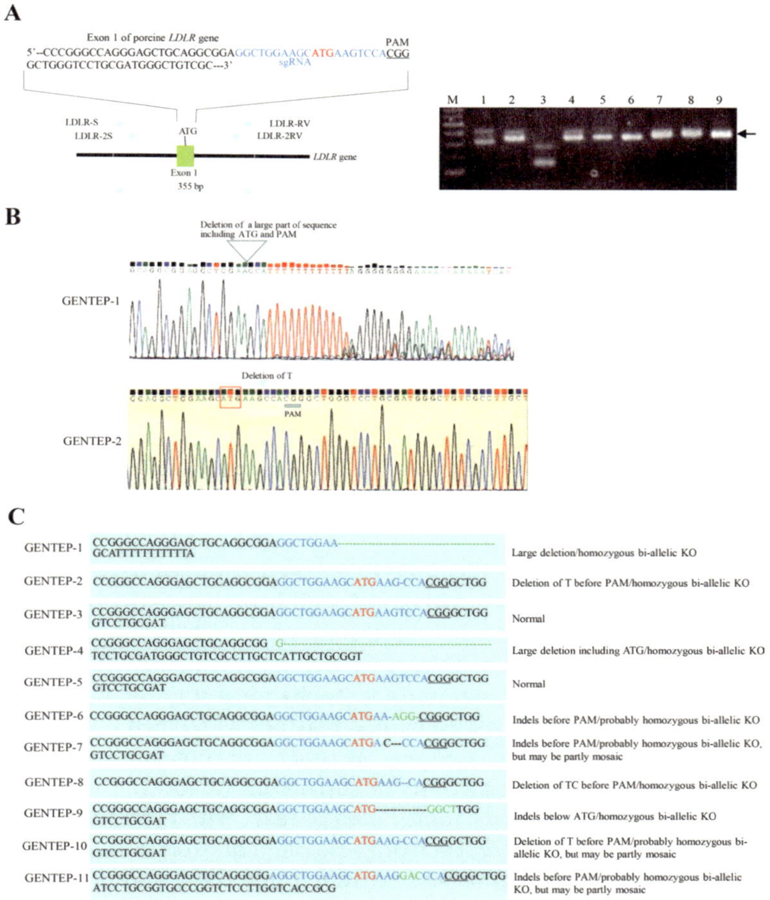

Figure 4.
Molecular biological analysis of the GENTEP-treated embryos (termed GENTEP-1 to -11) at a single embryo level. (A) Structure of porcine LDLR *gene and a target sequence recognized by sgRNA (left panel), and the results of nested PCR (right panel). The target sequence (shown in blue) spanning ATG (shown in red) is located on the first exon of* LDLR. *PAM, protospacer adjacent motif. Primers used for first PCR and nested PCR are shown above the* LDRL. *In the right panel, a part of the nested PCR products (lanes 1–9) loaded onto 2% agarose gel is shown. Arrow indicates the PCR products of 355 bp in size. M, 100-bp ladder markers. (B) Ideogram pattern in the GENTEP-1 and -2 samples obtained after direct sequencing of the nested PCR products using LDLR-2S primer. (C) Various indels found in each GENTEP-treated embryo. ATG is shown in red. Sequence recognized by sgRNA is shown in blue.*

first exon of porcine *LDLR* (left panel of **Figure 4A**). The sgRNA was synthesized by Integrated DNA Technologies, Inc. (IDT; Coralville, Iowa, USA) as Alt-R™ CRISPR crRNA product. The crRNA and tracrRNA (purchased from IDT) were combined for annealing and then mixed with recombinant Cas9 protein (TaKaRa Shuzo Co. Ltd., Shiga, Japan) to form RNP, according to the method of Ohtsuka et al. [139]. The final concentrations of the components in RNP were 30 μM/mL (for crRNA/tracrRNA) and 1 mg/mL (for Cas9 protein). The SCNT-treated embryos 6 or 12 h after activation were transferred to a 5-μL drop (containing RNP in Opti-MEM) and immediately subjected to *in vitro* EP under these conditions: 30 V, square pulses, 1.0 ms in duration at 99 ms intervals (or 0.5 ms in duration at 99.5 ms intervals), both repeated seven times. After EP, the embryos were promptly cultivated in normal medium for 7 days up to blastocysts and then subjected to analysis of molecular biology (possible mutations in the first exon of *LDLR*) and immunocytochemistry (possible loss of LDLR protein synthesis) parameters, as described

Stage at EP after activation of SCNT-treated embryos	EP condition[2]	Total number of SCNT-treated embryos examined	No. of embryos cleaved to the two-cell stage (%)	No. of embryos developed to blastocysts (%)
6 h	0.5	12	8 (66.7)	1 (8.3)
	1.0	12	11 (91.7)	2 (16.7)
12 h	0.5	33	21 (63.6)	5 (15.2)
	1.0	35	23 (65.7)	3 (8.6)

[1]*EP in the presence of RNP [10 μM of crRNA/tracrRNA mixture (targeted to LDLR gene) + 0.3 μg/μL of Cas9 protein] is performed on SCNT-treated embryos 6 or 12 h after activation. The EP-treated embryos were then cultured for 7 days to the blastocyst stage for the presence of mutations in the target gene at molecular biological and immunocytochemical levels.*
[2]*EP was performed under the electric condition of 30 V in voltage, 0.5 ms in length of square pulse with 99.5-ms intervals (0.5) or 1.0 ms in length of square pulse with 99-ms intervals (1.0), and seven times of pulse stimulation using an electroporation chamber (#LF610P4-4_470; BEX Co. Ltd.) connected to an electric pulse generator (CUY21EDITII. Genome Editor™, BEX Co. Ltd.).*

Table 2.
Summary of the properties of blastocysts derived from EP[1] toward the SCNT-treated porcine embryos.

in **Figure 2B**. In each group, 8–17% of the EP-treated embryos developed to blastocysts (**Table 2**). These rates appear to be comparable to the yield (24.2%) in experiments performed using intact MMP fetal fibroblasts as SCNT donors [119]. All of the blastocysts obtained were then fixed with 4% paraformaldehyde, and a section of these embryos was subjected to immunocytochemical staining using anti-LDLR antibody (**Figure 2B**). The EP-treated cloned blastocyst (termed GENTEP-1) was unreactive to anti-LDLR (arrows in **Figure 3B(g–i)**). In contrast, a parthenote (blastocyst) exhibited positive reactivity to anti-LDLR (arrow in **Figure 3B(a–c)**). Staining with the second antibody alone failed to react with the antibody (arrow in **Figure 3B(d–f)**). Furthermore, each of these fixed blastocysts was subjected to genomic DNA isolation to examine possible mutations at the individual embryo level (**Figure 2B**). Next, GenomiPhi-based whole genome amplification (WGA) was performed using the isolated genomic DNA as a template, as described previously [140]. PCR was then performed using the WGA products as a PCR template. The primer sets used are LDLR-S (5′-AAACCTCACATTGAAATGCTG-3′)/LDLR-RV (5′-CCTAAACTCTCGCGCCCCCCT-3′) for the first round of PCR and LDLR-2S (5′-CTGCAAATGACTGGGGCCCCG-3′)/LDLR-2RV (5′-CTCCAACCACGTAAGAATGAC-3′) for nested PCR (left panel of **Figure 4A**). Nested PCR using the LDLR-2S/LDLR-2RV primer set yields 355-bp products (left panel of **Figure 4A**). The typical example when the nested PCR products (lanes 1–9) are loaded onto a 2% agarose gel is shown in the right panel of **Figure 4A**. Almost all of the samples tested exhibited 355-bp products, except for lane 3 showing bands of reduced size, suggesting occurrence of a large deletion (probably over 100 bp) around the *LDLR* sequence recognized by sgRNA. In **Figure 4B**, an example of the results obtained from direct sequencing of nested PCR products using LDLR-2S primer is shown. The sample GENTEP-1, which has been shown to exhibit loss of the reactivity to anti-LDLR (see **Figure 3B-g-i**), had a large deletion including a sequence spanning ATG and PAM. Notably, there was no appreciable overlapping in ideograms of the sample, suggesting a homozygous bi-allelic KO phenotype (**Figure 4C**). Subcloning of the PCR products derived from the sample GENTEP-1 into TA cloning vector and subsequent sequencing demonstrated that all six clones obtained exhibited the same sequence as the parental product (data not shown). When the remaining PCR products were sequenced it was found that almost all (82%, 9/11) of the samples exhibited the homozygous bi-allelic KO genotype (**Figure 4C**).

5. Other techniques and factors affecting efficacy of the genome editing system

As shown above, genome editing tools such as ZFNs, TALENs and CRISPR/Cas9 are considered useful in enabling site-specific gene modification in livestock such as pigs. However, there are still several techniques and factors that influence performance which must be addressed. These include the single embryo assay, off-target cutting, multiplexed genome engineering, KI, and Cas9 pigs. In this section, these techniques or factors are described in greater detail.

5.1 Single embryo assay

To increasing the efficiency of genome editing systems, it is important to select suitable sets of ZFNs (or TALENs) or sgRNA (in the case of CRISPR/Cas9). Researchers therefore must check the efficiency of these reagents by introducing them into cultured cells, but at this point it remains unknown whether they will function *in vivo*. Unlike small animals such as mice and rats, large animals have long gestation periods and it is costly to prepare large animal recipients. Therefore, this testing *in vivo* appears to be difficult in larger animals such as pigs. To overcome this issue, a single embryo (blastocyst) assay to evaluate the operability of the genome editing reagents prepared was provided by Wang et al. [62] who later re-validated those sets using porcine parthenotes. To our knowledge, this assay was first developed using mice by Sakurai et al. [141] who reported that it is useful for confirming the fidelity of sgRNAs used.

It may be required to confirm at a molecular level whether the genome-edited embryos have mutations. In this case, WGA has often been employed for amplifying the whole genome of an embryo (blastocyst) using genomic DNA isolated from a single embryo as the DNA template [140, 141], since the blastocyst DNA is often too small to generate a sufficient amount of PCR product. The effectiveness of WGA-based amplification of blastocyst DNA has already been confirmed by ours [142] and others [44]. The resulting products obtained after PCR using WGA-derived DNA as the template are then subjected to direct sequencing for identification of possible mutations in the target gene, as shown in **Figure 4B**.

5.2 Off-target cleavage

Since sgRNA used in the CRISPR/Cas9 system can recognize only a short sequence (20 bp) at the target gene where Cas9 cleaves, other genes with a similar sequence to the sgRNA may be susceptible to Cas9-mediated DNA cleavage, which leads to the occasional generation of off-target cutting [29, 143]. This unintended cutting is considered a serious problem to be resolved.

Several strategies to minimize off-target cutting have been employed including the use of the double nickase mutant form of Cas9, which induces a single-strand break instead of DSB [144]; the use of RNP, whose half-life is shorter than the duration of transcription of plasmid or viral nucleic acids [110, 145]; or the fusion of catalytically inactive Cas9 with *Fok* I nuclease domain (fCas9) to improve the DNA cleavage specificity [146]. Recently, it was reported that Cpf1, a putative Class 2 CRISPR effector, mediates target DNA editing differently from Cas9 [147]. It generates a 5-nucleotide staggered cut with a 5′ overhang, which is particularly advantageous in facilitating an NHEJ-based KI into a genome. Several unique enzymes that can decrease the probability of off-target cleavage have also been produced. For example, two engineered enzymes produced from SpCas9 from *Streptococcus pyogenes* with the goal of enhancing specificity, called eSpCas9 [148] and SpCas9-HF [149], are reported to reduce the probability of mismatched DNA binding. A hybrid enzyme combining the Cas9-nickase and PmCDA1, an activation-induced cytidine deaminase (AID) ortholog, could perform targeted nucleotide substitution [150]. Furthermore, a CRISPR system using a new Cas-related enzyme called Cas13a that targets RNA has also been recently developed [151].

Notably, in the case of GE pigs and embryos, there have been no reports of off-target mutagenesis as shown by the following papers: [43, 50, 61–64, 69, 74, 77, 78, 80, 86, 100, 105]. This suggests a very low probability of off target-cleavage in GE pigs.

5.3 Multiplexed genome engineering

The CRISPR/Cas9 system can confer multigene KO in one shot of gene delivery [152, 153]. This property is especially beneficial for the purpose of creating disease model animals, as certain types of diseases are known to be caused by multigene defects. Interestingly, Sakurai et al. [154] demonstrated that at least nine endogenous genes can be knocked out simultaneously through a single shot of cytoplasmic MI of 12 sgRNAs together with Cas9 mRNA into murine zygotes. In pigs, Zhou et al. [61] demonstrated successful generation of PARK2 (*parkin*) and PTEN-induced putative kinase 1 (*PINK1*) double-KO pigs through SCNT with GE fetal fibroblasts after co-transfection of Cas9, *PARK2*-sgRNA, and *PINK1*-sgRNA-expressing vectors by electroporation. The percentage of $PARK2^{-/-}/PINK1^{-/-}$ double-KO cells was up to 38.1%. SCNT using these double-KO cells resulted in the birth of 20 cloned piglets. Of these, four piglets developed normally, and both parkin and PINK1 in those individuals were depleted at the protein level. Estrada et al. [66] also succeeded in obtaining one triple-KO cloned piglet with mutations in *GGTA1* (coding for α-1,3-galactosyltransferase), *CMAH* (coding for cytidine monophosphate-*N*-acetylneuraminic acid hydroxylase) and *β4GalNT2* (coding for β1,4-*N*-acetylgalactosaminyl transferase) after SCNT. Wang et al. [81] generated PARK7 (*DJ-1*)/*parkin*/*PINK1* triple-gene modified pigs using the CRISPR/Cas9 system in one step through direct zygote injection of Cas9 mRNA and three types of sgRNAs. According to Wang et al. [81], of two live-born piglets delivered, one piglet showed biallelic modification of all three genes, and another showed biallelic modification of the *DJ-1* and *PINK1* genes and monoallelic mutation of the *parkin* gene.

5.4 KI

As shown in **Table 1**, in 2015 successful KI in pigs was reported by several groups. For example, Wang et al. [62] performed MI with *in vivo* fertilized zygotes (derived from colored pigs) using Cas9 mRNA + sgRNA + single-stranded DNA oligonucleotides (ssODN), targeting microphthalmia-associated transcription factor (MITF), a master regulator gene of melanocyte development, and obtained two live-born piglets showing the white coat color phenotype over its entire body. Peng et al. [63] tried to create KI piglets with a MI approach using a circular vector as donor DNA. They designed an sgRNA targeting the starting codon region (including the adjacent 5′ and ATG) and generated a targeted fragment (donor for HR) with the insert flanked by 1-kb HA on both sides. They performed cytoplasmic MI of Cas9 mRNA + *in vitro* synthesized sgRNA + circular vector containing the targeting fragment, and finally obtained 16 live piglets, all of which were found to carry the expected KI allele. Notably, they confirmed expression of human albumin (Alb) protein generated from the KI allele in the plasma of these cloned pigs. This means that expression of a transgene (human Alb as GOI) is possible under the control of an endogenous promoter system (in this case, Alb promoter).

Ruan et al. [60] demonstrated production of GE pigs with successful KI of GOI into the target *Hipp11* (*H11*) locus, which is considered as "safe harbor" genomic locus that allows gene expression without disrupting internal gene function, like the *Rosa26* locus. They utilized a positive and negative selection method to insert *GFP* into the *pH 11* locus in pig fetal fibroblast cells by electroporation. The targeting donor vector (4.2 kb in size) contains a reporter cassette with *neo* and GFP genes which are flanked by a 0.8-kb HA to the *H11* locus on each side with the diphtheria toxin A (DTA) gene at the 3′ end. Cells were transfected with the linearized donor vector and two expression vectors for sgRNA (targeted to the *H11* locus) and Cas9. After drug selection, they obtained GE cells with successful KI at the *H11* locus with efficiencies up to 54%. Next, they performed SCNT using these correctly targeted clones, and obtained one cloned piglet which was later confirmed to show correct targeting.

Generally, it is believed that HDR-mediated KI is more difficult than NHEJ-based indels. For example, in proliferating human cells, NHEJ has been reported to repair 75% of DSBs, while HDR repaired the remaining 25% [155]. To enhance the HDR efficiency, several approaches are now being attempted. For examples, co-injection of murine zygotes with a mixture containing Cas9 mRNA, sgRNA, template ssODNs and Scr7 (an inhibitor for DNA ligase IV) significantly improved the efficiency of HDR-mediated insertional mutagenesis [156]. Chu et al. [157] also demonstrated usefulness of Scr7 for abolishing NHEJ activity and increasing HDR in both human and mouse cell lines. However, the function of Scr7 in promoting HDR remains controversial. Some researchers demonstrated that Scr7 failed to increase HDR rates in rabbit embryos [158] and porcine fetal fibroblasts [159]. On the contrary, Li et al. [160] demonstrated that Scr7 promoted HDR efficiency in porcine fetal fibroblasts. The same group also showed that other reagents L755507 (β-3 adrenergic receptor agonist) and resveratrol (small-molecule compound found in grapes) also showed similar effects (promotion of HDR efficiency) in porcine cells.

5.5 Cas9 pigs

As mentioned previously, the current generation of gene-edited pigs has mostly been produced through either MI or SCNT approaches, which are both expensive and time-consuming. In mice, several Tg lines carrying a Cas9-expressing cassette have been created [154, 161, 162]. These Tg mice are thought to be useful animals for direct *in vivo* genome editing experiments, because successful delivery of the expression vectors of sgRNAs alone or RNA itself into selected tissues caused generation of genome-edited tissues. For example, Platt et al. [161] demonstrated that *in vivo* viral administration of Kirsten rat sarcoma viral oncogene homolog (*Kras*), transformation related protein 53 (*Trp53*), and serine/threonine-protein kinase 11 (*Stk11*)-gRNAs to the Cas9-expressing line caused lung carcinomas within a short period. This suggests that if a Cas9-expressing pig is produced, it will provide an easy and efficient way to produce genetic modifications, which should substantially facilitate studying gene functions, modeling human diseases, and promoting agricultural productivity. Based on this concept, Wang et al. [163] first produced Cre-dependent Cas9-expressing pigs to enable efficient *in vivo* genome editing. They first transfected the linear-targeting donor containing Cre-dependent Cas9-expression cassette and TALEN plasmids directed to *Rosa26* locus into porcine fetal fibroblasts and finally selected clones carrying KI cassette. These clones were then used for SCNT to produce cloned GE piglets. They showed that cells isolated from several organs of GE pigs exhibited Cre-induced activation of Cas9 expression. This Cas9 pig line will be used for various studies as indicated above.

6. Conclusion

Because pigs are similar to humans in physiological, anatomical, and genetic aspects, they are now seen as a leading animal model for biomedical research. Recent advances in genome editing technology have led to accelerated production of GE pigs within a relatively short time period, which is beneficial due to cost savings in propagation of GE animals and maintaining animals for breeding. Production of GE pigs can be largely categorized into two approaches, so-called MI/EP-mediated production of GE zygotes and SCNT using GE cells as the SCNT donor. There are advantages and drawbacks for both these approaches. For example, the former is simpler, more convenient, and cost-effective than the latter. However, the available genetic background is limited. In this context, the latter is beneficial for the flexibility of choosing any type of genetic background, because the genetic background of SCNT-derived cloned pigs is determined by that of donor cells used for SCNT. Unfortunately, the efficiency of SCNT is extremely low at present. MI/EP with SCNT-treated embryos may compensate for these disadvantages associated with MI/EP or SCNT-mediated production of GE piglets, if the efficiency of SCNT is greatly improved in future.

Acknowledgements

We thank Shogo Matsunaga for their support in the GENTEP-related experiment, shown in **Figures 3** and **4**. This study was partly supported by a grant (no. 19K06372 for Masahiro Sato; nos. 25450475 and 16K08085 for Kazuchika Miyoshi; no. 18K09839 for Emi Inada; no. 17H04412 for Issei Saitoh; no. 16H05176 for Akihide Tanimoto) from the Ministry of Education, Science, Sports, and Culture, Japan.

Conflicts of interest

The founding sponsors had no role in the design of the study, collection, analyses, or interpretation of data, writing of the manuscript, and decision to publish the results.

Author contributions

Masahiro Sato designed the study and drafted the manuscript; Kazuchika Miyoshi and Hiroaki Kawaguchi involved in the GENTEP-related experiment; Emi Inada and Issei Saitoh critically revised the manuscript; Akihide Tanimoto supervised the manuscript.

Author details

Masahiro Sato[1]*, Kazuchika Miyoshi[2], Hiroaki Kawaguchi[3], Emi Inada[4], Issei Saitoh[5] and Akihide Tanimoto[6]

1 Section of Gene Expression Regulation, Frontier Science Research Center, Kagoshima University, Kagoshima, Japan

2 Laboratory of Animal Reproduction, Faculty of Agriculture, Kagoshima University, Kagoshima, Japan

3 Department of Hygiene and Health Promotion Medicine, Graduate School of Medical and Dental Sciences, Kagoshima University, Kagoshima, Japan

4 Department of Pediatric Dentistry, Graduate School of Medical and Dental Sciences, Kagoshima University, Kagoshima, Japan

5 Division of Pediatric Dentistry, Graduate School of Medical and Dental Science, Niigata University, Niigata, Japan

6 Department of Pathology, Division of Oncology, Graduate School of Medical and Dental Sciences, Kagoshima University, Kagoshima, Japan

*Address all correspondence to: masasato@m.kufm.kagoshima-u.ac.jp

References

[1] Cooper DKC, Gollackner B, Sachs DH. Will the pig solve the transplantation backlog? Annual Review of Medicine. 2002;**53**:133-147. DOI: 10.1146/annurev.med.53.082901.103900

[2] Fan N, Lai L. Genetically modified pig models for human diseases. Journal of Genetics and Genomics. 2013;**40**: 67-73. DOI: 10.1016/j.jgg.2012.07.014

[3] Yang H, Wu Z. Genome editing of pigs for agriculture and biomedicine. Frontiers in Genetics. 2018;**9**:360. DOI: 10.3389/fgene.2018.00360

[4] Gordon JW, Scangos GA, Plotkin DJ, Barbosa JA, Ruddle FH. Genetic transformation of mouse embryos by microinjection of purified DNA. Proceedings of the National Academy of Sciences of the United States of America. 1980;**77**:7380-7384. DOI: 10.1073/pnas.77.12.7380

[5] Hammer RE, Pursel VG, Rexroad CE Jr, Wall RJ, Bolt DJ, et al. Production of transgenic rabbits, sheep and pigs by microinjection. Nature. 1985;**315**: 680-683. DOI: 10.1038/315680a0

[6] Bestor TH, Chandler VL, Feinberg AP. Epigenetic effects in eukaryotic gene expression. Developmental Genetics. 1994;**15**:458-462. DOI: 10.1002/dvg.1020150603

[7] Doetschman T, Gregg RG, Maeda N, Hooper ML, Melton DW, et al. Targetted correction of a mutant HPRT gene in mouse embryonic stem cells. Nature. 1987;**330**:576-578. DOI: 10.1038/330576a0

[8] Bouabe H, Okkenhaug K. Gene targeting in mice: A review. Methods in Molecular Biology. 2013;**1064**:315-336. DOI: 10.1007/978-1-62703-601-6_23

[9] Notarianni E, Galli C, Laurie S, Moor RM, Evans MJ. Derivation of pluripotent, embryonic cell lines from the pig and sheep. Journal of Reproduction and Fertility. Supplement. 1991;**43**:255-260

[10] Chen LR, Shiue YL, Bertolini L, Medrano JF, BonDurant RH, et al. Establishment of pluripotent cell lines from porcine preimplantation embryos. Theriogenology. 1999;**52**:195-212. DOI: 10.1016/S0093-691X(99)00122-3

[11] Ezashi T, Telugu BP, Alexenko AP, Sachdev S, Sinha S, et al. Derivation of induced pluripotent stem cells from pig somatic cells. Proceedings of the National Academy of Sciences of the United States of America. 2009;**106**:10993-10998. DOI: 10.1073/pnas.0905284106

[12] Brevini TA, Pennarossa G, Gandolfi F. No shortcuts to pig embryonic stem cells. Theriogenology. 2010;**74**:544-550. DOI: 10.1016/j.theriogenology.2010.04.020

[13] Hou DR, Jin Y, Nie XW, Zhang ML, Ta N, et al. Derivation of porcine embryonic stem-like cells from *in vitro*-produced blastocyst-stage embryos. Scientific Reports. 2016;**6**:25838. DOI: 10.1038/srep25838

[14] Campbell KH, McWhir J, Ritchie WA, Wilmut I. Sheep cloned by nuclear transfer from a cultured cell line. Nature. 1996;**380**:64-66. DOI: 10.1038/380064a0

[15] Wilmut I, Schnieke AE, McWhir J, Kind AJ, Campbell KH. Viable offspring derived from fetal and adult mammalian cells. Nature. 1997;**385**:810-813. DOI: 10.1038/385810a0

[16] Prather RS, Sims MM, First NL. Nuclear transplantation in early pig embryos. Biology of Reproduction. 1989;**41**:414-418. DOI: 10.1095/biolreprod41.3.414

[17] Schnieke AE, Kind AJ, Ritchie WA, Mycock K, Scott AR, et al. Human factor IX transgenic sheep produced by transfer of nuclei from transfected fetal fibroblasts. Science. 1997;**278**:2130-2133. DOI: 10.1126/science.278.5346.2130

[18] Denning C, Burl S, Ainslie A, Bracken J, Dinnyes A, et al. Deletion of the alpha(1,3)galactosyl transferase (GGTA1) gene and the prion protein (PrP) gene in sheep. Nature Biotechnology. 2001;**19**:559-562. DOI: 10.1038/89313

[19] Polejaeva IA, Chen SH, Vaught TD, Page RL, Mullins J, et al. Cloned pigs produced by nuclear transfer from adult somatic cells. Nature. 2000;**407**:86-90. DOI: 10.1038/35024082

[20] Sachs DH, Galli C. Genetic manipulation in pigs. Current Opinion in Organ Transplantation. 2009;**14**:148-153. DOI: 10.1097/MOT.0b013e3283292549

[21] Wells KD, Prather RS. Genome-editing technologies to improve research, reproduction, and production in pigs. Molecular Reproduction and Development. 2017;**84**:1012-1017. DOI: 10.1002/mrd.22812

[22] Park KW, Cheong HT, Lai L, Im GS, Kühholzer B, et al. Production of nuclear transfer-derived swine that express the enhanced green fluorescent protein. Animal Biotechnology. 2001;**12**:173-181. DOI: 10.1081/ABIO-100108344

[23] Lai L, Kolber-Simonds D, Park KW, Cheong HT, Greenstein JL, et al. Production of alpha-1,3-galactosyltransferase knockout pigs by nuclear transfer cloning. Science. 2002;**295**:1089-1092. DOI: 10.1126/science.1068228

[24] Dai Y, Vaught TD, Boone J, Chen SH, Phelps CJ, et al. Targeted disruption of the alpha1,3-galactosyltransferase gene in cloned pigs. Nature Biotechnology. 2002;**20**:251-255. DOI: 10.1038/nbt0302-251

[25] Lai LX, Kang JX, Li RF, Wang JD, Witt WT, et al. Generation of cloned transgenic pigs rich in omega-3 fatty acids. Nature Biotechnology. 2006;**24**:435-436. DOI: 10.1038/nbt1198

[26] Rogers CS, Stoltz DA, Meyerholz DK, Ostedgaard LS, Rokhlina T, et al. Disruption of the CFTR gene produces a model of cystic fibrosis in newborn pigs. Science. 2008;**321**:1837-1841. DOI: 10.1126/science.1163600

[27] Suzuki S, Iwamoto M, Saito Y, Fuchimoto D, Sembon S, et al. Il2rg gene-targeted severe combined immunodeficiency pigs. Cell Stem Cell. 2012;**10**:753-758. DOI: 10.1016/j.stem.2012.04.021

[28] Tan W, Proudfoot C, Lillico SG, Whitelaw CB. Gene targeting, genome editing: From Dolly to editors. Transgenic Research. 2016;**25**:273-287. DOI: 10.1007/s11248-016-9932-x

[29] Hsu PD, Lander ES, Zhang F. Development and applications of CRISPR-Cas9 for genome engineering. Cell. 2014;**157**:1262-1278. DOI: 10.1016/j.cell.2014.05.010

[30] Sonoda E, Hochegger H, Saberi A, Taniguchi Y, Takeda S. Differential usage of non-homologous end-joining and homologous recombination in double strand break repair. DNA Repair. 2006;**5**:1021-1029. DOI: 10.1016/j.dnarep.2006.05.022

[31] Kim YG, Cha J, Chandrasegaran S. Hybrid restriction enzymes: Zinc finger fusions to Fok I cleavage domain. Proceedings of the National Academy of Sciences of the United States of America. 1996;**93**:1156-1160. DOI: 10.1073/pnas.93.3.1156

[32] Urnov FD, Miller JC, Lee YL, Beausejour CM, Rock JM, et al. Highly efficient endogenous human gene correction using designed zinc-finger

nucleases. Nature. 2005;**435**:646-651. DOI: 10.1038/nature03556

[33] Christian M, Cermak T, Doyle EL, Schmidt C, Zhang F, et al. Targeting DNA double-strand breaks with TAL effector nucleases. Genetics. 2010;**186**:757-761. DOI: 10.1534/genetics.110.120717

[34] Miller JC, Tan S, Qiao G, Barlow KA, Wang J, et al. A TALE nuclease architecture for efficient genome editing. Nature Biotechnology. 2011;**29**:143-148. DOI: 10.1038/nbt.1755

[35] Reyon D, Tsai SQ, Khayter C, Foden JA, Sander JD, et al. FLASH assembly of TALENs for high-throughput genome editing. Nature Biotechnology. 2012;**30**:460-465. DOI: 10.1038/nbt.2170

[36] Cermak T, Doyle EL, Christian M, Wang L, Zhang Y, et al. Efficient design and assembly of custom TALEN and other TAL effector-based constructs for DNA targeting. Nucleic Acids Research. 2011;**39**:e82. DOI: 10.1093/nar/gkr218

[37] Horvath P, Barrangou R. CRISPR/Cas, the immune system of bacteria and archaea. Science. 2010;**327**:167-170. DOI: 10.1126/science.1179555

[38] Bhaya D, Davison M, Barrangou R. CRISPR-Cas systems in bacteria and archaea: Versatile small RNAs for adaptive defense and regulation. Annual Review of Genetics. 2011;**45**:273-297. DOI: 10.1146/annurev-genet-110410-132430

[39] Jinek M, Chylinski K, Fonfara I, Hauer M, Doudna JA, et al. A programmable dual-RNA-guided DNA endonuclease in adaptive bacterial immunity. Science. 2012;**337**:816-821. DOI: 10.1126/science.1225829

[40] Gaj T, Gersbach CA, Barbas CFIII. ZFN, TALEN, and CRISPR/Cas-based methods for genome engineering. Trends in Biotechnology. 2013;**31**:397-405. DOI: 10.1016/j.tibtech.2013.04.004

[41] Whyte JJ, Zhao J, Wells KD, Samuel MS, Whitworth KM, et al. Gene targeting with zinc finger nucleases to produce cloned eGFP knockout pigs. Molecular Reproduction and Development. 2011;**78**:2. DOI: 10.1002/mrd.21271

[42] Yang D, Yang H, Li W, Zhao B, Ouyang Z, et al. Generation of PPARgamma mono-allelic knockout pigs via zinc-finger nucleases and nuclear transfer cloning. Cell Research. 2011;**21**:979-982. DOI: 10.1038/cr.2011.70

[43] Hauschild J, Petersen B, Santiago Y, Queisser AL, Carnwath JW, et al. Efficient generation of a biallelic knockout in pigs using zinc-finger nucleases. Proceedings of the National Academy of Sciences of the United States of America. 2011;**108**:12013-12017. DOI: 10.1073/pnas.1106422108

[44] Carlson DF, Tan W, Lillico SG, Stverakova D, Proudfoot C, et al. Efficient TALEN-mediated gene knockout in livestock. Proceedings of the National Academy of Sciences of the United States of America. 2012;**109**:17382-17387. DOI: 10.1073/pnas.1211446109

[45] Lillico SG, Proudfoot C, Carlson DF, Stverakova D, Neil C, et al. Live pigs produced from genome edited zygotes. Scientific Reports. 2013;**3**:2847. DOI: 10.1038/srep02847

[46] Xin J, Yang H, Fan N, Zhao B, Ouyang Z, et al. Highly efficient generation of GGTA1 biallelic knockout inbred mini-pigs with TALENs. PLoS ONE. 2013;**8**:e84250. DOI: 10.1371/journal.pone.0084250

[47] Tan W, Carlson DF, Lancto CA, Garbe JR, Webster DA, et al. Efficient nonmeiotic allele introgression in

livestock using custom endonucleases. Proceedings of the National Academy of Sciences of the United States of America. 2013;**110**:16526-16531. DOI: 10.1073/pnas.1310478110

[48] Watanabe M, Nakano K, Matsunari H, Matsuda T, Maehara M, et al. Generation of interleukin-2 receptor gamma gene knockout pigs from somatic cells genetically modified by zinc finger nuclease-encoding mRNA. PLoS ONE. 2013;**8**:e76478. DOI: 10.1371/journal.pone.0076478

[49] Lutz AJ, Li P, Estrada JL, Sidner RA, Chihara RK, et al. Double knockout pigs deficient in N-glycolylneuraminic acid and galactose alpha-1,3-galactose reduce the humoral barrier to xenotransplantation. Xenotransplantation. 2013;**20**:27-35. DOI: 10.1111/xen.12019

[50] Kwon DN, Lee K, Kang MJ, Choi YJ, Park C, et al. Production of biallelic CMP-Neu5Ac hydroxylase knock-out pigs. Scientific Reports. 2013;**3**:1981. DOI: 10.1038/srep01981

[51] Whitworth KM, Lee K, Benne JA, Beaton BP, Spate LD, et al. CRISPR/Cas9 system to produce genetically engineered pigs from *in vitro*-derived oocytes and embryos. Biology of Reproduction. 2014;**91**:78. DOI: 10.1095/biolreprod.114.121723

[52] Hai T, Teng F, Guo R, Li W, Zhou Q. One-step generation of knockout pigs by zygote injection of CRISPR/Cas system. Cell Research. 2014;**24**:372-375. DOI: 10.1038/cr.2014.11

[53] Reyes LM, Estrada JL, Wang ZY, Blosser RJ, Smith RF, et al. Creating class I MHC-null pigs using guide RNA and the Cas9 endonuclease. Journal of Immunology. 2014;**193**:5751-5757. DOI: 10.4049/jimmunol.1402059

[54] Huang J, Guo X, Fan N, Song J, Zhao B, et al. RAG1/2 knockout pigs with severe combined immunodeficiency. Journal of Immunology. 2014;**193**: 1496-1503. DOI: 10.4049/jimmunol.1400915

[55] Bao L, Chen H, Jong U, Rim C, Li W, et al. Generation of GGTA1 biallelic knockout pigs via zinc-finger nucleases and somatic cell nuclear transfer. Science China. Life Sciences. 2014;**57**:263-268. DOI: 10.1007/s11427-013-4601-2

[56] Li P, Estrada JL, Burlak C, Montgomery J, Butler JR, et al. Efficient generation of genetically distinct pigs in a single pregnancy using multiplexed single-guide RNA and carbohydrate selection. Xenotransplantation. 2015;**22**:20-31. DOI: 10.1111/xen.12131

[57] Qian L, Tang M, Yang J, Wang Q, Cai C, et al. Targeted mutations in myostatin by zinc-finger nucleases result in double-muscled phenotype in Meishan pigs. Scientific Reports. 2015;**5**:14435. DOI: 10.1038/srep14435

[58] Paris LL, Estrada JL, Li P, Blankenship RL, Sidner RA, et al. Reduced human platelet uptake by pig livers deficient in the asialoglycoprotein receptor 1 protein. Xenotransplantation. 2015;**22**:203-210. DOI: 10.1111/xen.12164

[59] Miyagawa S, Matsunari H, Watanabe M, Nakano K, Umeyama K, et al. Generation of alpha1,3-galactosyltransferase and cytidine monophospho-N-acetylneuraminic acid hydroxylase gene double-knockout pigs. Journal of Reproduction and Development. 2015;**61**:449-457. DOI: 10.1262/jrd.2015-058

[60] Ruan J, Li H, Xu K, Wu T, Wei J, et al. Highly efficient CRISPR/Cas9-mediated transgene knockin at the H11 locus in pigs. Scientific Reports. 2015;**5**:14253. DOI: 10.1038/srep14253

[61] Zhou X, Xin J, Fan N, Zou Q, Huang J, et al. Generation of CRISPR/

Cas9-mediated gene-targeted pigs via somatic cell nuclear transfer. Cellular and Molecular Life Sciences. 2015;**72**:1175-1184. DOI: 10.1007/s00018-014-1744-7

[62] Wang X, Zhou J, Cao C, Huang J, Hai T, et al. Efficient CRISPR/Cas9-mediated biallelic gene disruption and site-specific knockin after rapid selection of highly active sgRNAs in pigs. Scientific Reports. 2015;**5**:13348. DOI: 10.1038/srep13348

[63] Peng J, Wang Y, Jiang J, Zhou X, Song L, et al. Production of human albumin in pigs through CRISPR/Cas9-mediated knockin of human cDNA into swine albumin locus in the zygotes. Scientific Reports. 2015;**5**:16705. DOI: 10.1038/srep16705

[64] Wang Y, Du Y, Shen B, Zhou X, Li J, et al. Efficient generation of gene-modified pigs via injection of zygote with Cas9/sgRNA. Scientific Reports. 2015;**5**:8256. DOI: 10.1038/srep08256

[65] Wang K, Ouyang H, Xie Z, Yao C, Guo N, et al. Efficient generation of myostatin mutations in pigs using the CRISPR/Cas9 system. Scientific Reports. 2015;**5**:16623. DOI: 10.1038/srep16623

[66] Estrada JL, Martens G, Li P, Adams A, Newell KA, et al. Evaluation of human and non-human primate antibody binding to pig cells lacking GGTA1/CMAH/β4GalNT2 genes. Xenotransplantation. 2015;**22**:194-202. DOI: 10.1111/xen.12161

[67] Chen F, Wang Y, Yuan Y, Zhang W, Ren Z, et al. Generation of B cell-deficient pigs by highly efficient CRISPR/Cas9-mediated gene targeting. Journal of Genetics and Genomics. 2015;**42**:437-444. DOI: 10.1016/j.jgg.2015.05.002

[68] Tanihara F, Takemoto T, Kitagawa E, Rao S, Do LT, et al. Somatic cell reprogramming-free generation of genetically modified pigs. Science Advances. 2016;**2**:e1600803. DOI: 10.1126/sciadv.1600803

[69] Yu HH, Zhao H, Qing YB, Pan WR, Jia BY, et al. Porcine zygote injection with Cas9/sgRNA results in DMD-modified pig with muscle dystrophy. International Journal of Molecular Sciences. 2016;**17**:E1668. DOI: 10.3390/ijms17101668

[70] Umeyama K, Watanabe K, Watanabe M, Horiuchi K, Nakano K, et al. Generation of heterozygous fibrillin-1 mutant cloned pigs from genome-edited foetal fibroblasts. Scientific Reports. 2016;**6**:24413. DOI: 10.1038/srep24413

[71] Bi Y, Hua Z, Liu X, Hua W, Ren H, et al. Isozygous and selectable marker-free MSTN knockout cloned pigs generated by the combined use of CRISPR/Cas9 and Cre/LoxP. Scientific Reports. 2016;**6**:31729. DOI: 10.1038/srep31729

[72] Cheng W, Zhao H, Yu H, Xin J, Wang J, et al. Efficient generation of GGTA1-null Diannan miniature pigs using TALENs combined with somatic cell nuclear transfer. Reproductive Biology and Endocrinology. 2016;**14**:77. DOI: 10.1186/s12958-016-0212-7

[73] Kang JT, Kwon DK, Park AR, Lee EJ, Yun YJ, et al. Production of alpha1,3-galactosyltransferase targeted pigs using transcription activator-like effector nuclease-mediated genome editing technology. Journal of Veterinary Science. 2016;**17**:89-96. DOI: 10.4142/jvs.2016.17.1.89

[74] Kang JT, Ryu J, Cho B, Lee EJ, Yun YJ, et al. Generation of RUNX3 knockout pigs using CRISPR/Cas9-mediated gene targeting. Reproduction in Domestic Animals. 2016;**51**:970-978. DOI: 10.1111/rda.12775

[75] Rao S, Fujimura T, Matsunari H, Sakuma T, Nakano K, et al. Efficient modification of the myostatin gene in

porcine somatic cells and generation of knockout piglets. Molecular Reproduction and Development. 2016;**83**:61-70. DOI: 10.1002/mrd.22591

[76] Yang Y, Wang K, Wu H, Jin Q, Ruan D, et al. Genetically humanized pigs exclusively expressing human insulin are generated through custom endonuclease-mediated seamless engineering. Journal of Molecular Cell Biology. 2016;**8**:174-177. DOI: 10.1093/jmcb/mjw008

[77] Wang K, Tang X, Liu Y, Xie Z, Zou X, et al. Efficient generation of orthologous point mutations in pigs via CRISPR-assisted ssODN-mediated homology-directed repair. Molecular Therapy—Nucleic Acids. 2016;**5**:**e396**. DOI: 10.1038/mtna.2016.101

[78] Feng C, Li X, Cui H, Long C, Liu X, et al. Highly efficient generation of GGTA1 knockout pigs using a combination of TALEN mRNA and magnetic beads with somatic cell nuclear transfer. Journal of Integrative Agriculture. 2016;**15**:1540-1549. DOI: 10.1016/S2095-3119(16)61347-3

[79] Zhou X, Wang L, Du Y, Xie F, Li L, et al. Efficient generation of gene-modified pigs harboring precise orthologous human mutation via CRISPR/Cas9-induced homology-directed repair in zygotes. Human Mutation. 2016;**37**:110-118. DOI: 10.1002/humu.22913

[80] Petersen B, Frenzel A, Lucas-Hahn A, Herrmann D, Hassel P, et al. Efficient production of biallelic GGTA1 knockout pigs by cytoplasmic microinjection of CRISPR/Cas9 into zygotes. Xenotransplantation. 2016;**23**:338-346. DOI: 10.1111/xen.12258

[81] Wang X, Cao C, Huang J, Yao J, Hai T, et al. One-step generation of triple gene-targeted pigs using CRISPR/Cas9 system. Scientific Reports. 2016;**6**:20620. DOI: 10.1038/srep20620

[82] Sheets TP, Park CH, Park KE, Powell A, Donovan DM, et al. Somatic cell nuclear transfer followed by CRIPSR/Cas9 microinjection results in highly efficient genome editing in cloned pigs. International Journal of Molecular Sciences. 2016;**17**:2031. DOI: 10.3390/ijms17122031

[83] Fischer K, Kraner-Scheiber S, Petersen B, Rieblinger B, Buermann A, et al. Efficient production of multi-modified pigs for xenotransplantation by 'combineering', gene stacking and gene editing. Scientific Reports. 2016;**6**:29081. DOI: 10.1038/srep29081

[84] Lei S, Ryu J, Wen K, Twitchell E, Bui T, et al. Increased and prolonged human norovirus infection in RAG2/IL2RG deficient gnotobiotic pigs with severe combined immunodeficiency. Scientific Reports. 2016;**6**:25222. DOI: 10.1038/srep25222

[85] Park KE, Kaucher AV, Powell A, Waqas MS, Sandmaier SE, et al. Generation of germline ablated male pigs by CRISPR/Cas9 editing of the NANOS2 gene. Scientific Reports. 2017;**7**:40176. DOI: 10.1038/srep40176

[86] Huang L, Hua Z, Xiao H, Cheng Y, Xu K, et al. CRISPR/Cas9-mediated ApoE$^{-/-}$ and LDLR$^{-/-}$ double gene knockout in pigs elevates serum LDL-C and TC levels. Oncotarget. 2017;**8**:37751-37760. DOI: 10.18632/oncotarget.1715

[87] Shen Y, Xu K, Yuan Z, Guo J, Zhao H, et al. Efficient generation of P53 biallelic knockout Diannan miniature pigs via TALENs and somatic cell nuclear transfer. Journal of Translational Medicine. 2017;**15**:224. DOI: 10.1186/s12967-017-1327-0

[88] Kang J, Kim S, Zhu H, Jin L, Guo Q, et al. Generation of cloned adult muscular pigs with myostatin gene mutation by genetic engineering. RSC Advances. 2017;**7**:12541-12549. DOI: 10.1039/C6RA28579A

[89] Niu D, Wei HJ, Lin L, George H, Wang T, et al. Inactivation of porcine endogenous retrovirus in pigs using CRISPR-Cas9. Science. 2017;**357**: 1303-1307. DOI: 10.1126/science.aan4187

[90] Wang K, Tang X, Xie Z, Zou X, Li M, et al. CRISPR/Cas9-mediated knockout of myostatin in Chinese indigenous Erhualian pigs. Transgenic Research. 2017;**26**:799-805. DOI: 10.1007/s11248-017-0044-z

[91] Zheng Q, Lin J, Huang J, Zhang H, Zhang R, et al. Reconstitution of UCP1 using CRISPR/Cas9 in the white adipose tissue of pigs decreases fat deposition and improves thermogenic capacity. Proceedings of the National Academy of Sciences of the United States of America. 2017;**114**:E9474-E9482. DOI: 10.1073/pnas.1707853114

[92] Park KE, Powell A, Sandmaier SE, Kim CM, Mileham A, et al. Targeted gene knock-in by CRISPR/Cas ribonucleoproteins in porcine zygotes. Scientific Reports. 2017;7:42458. DOI: 10.1038/srep42458

[93] Whitworth KM, Benne JA, Spate LD, Murphy SL, Samuel MS, et al. Zygote injection of CRISPR/Cas9 RNA successfully modifies the target gene without delaying blastocyst development or altering the sex ratio in pigs. Transgenic Research. 2017;**26**: 97-107. DOI: 10.1007/s11248-016-9989-6

[94] Chuang CK, Chen CH, Huang CL, Su YH, Peng SH, et al. Generation of GGTA1 mutant pigs by direct pronuclear microinjection of CRISPR/Cas9 plasmid vectors. Animal Biotechnology. 2017;**28**:174-181. DOI: 10.1080/10495398.2016.1246453

[95] Wu J, Vilarino M, Suzuki K, Okamura D, Bogliotti YS, et al. CRISPR-Cas9 mediated one-step disabling of pancreatogenesis in pigs. Scientific Reports. 2017;7:10487. DOI: 10.1038/s41598-017-08596-5

[96] Gao H, Zhao C, Xiang X, Li Y, Zhao Y, et al. Production of α1,3-galactosyltransferase and cytidine monophosphate-N-acetylneuraminic acid hydroxylase gene double-deficient pigs by CRISPR/Cas9 and handmade cloning. Journal of Reproduction and Development. 2017;**63**:17-26. DOI: 10.1262/jrd.2016-079

[97] Tanihara F, Hirata M, Nguyen NT, Le QA, Hirano T, et al. Generation of a TP53-modified porcine cancer model by CRISPR/Cas9-mediated gene modification in porcine zygotes via electroporation. PLoS ONE. 2018;**13**:e0206360. DOI: 10.1371/journal.pone.0206360

[98] Li M, Ouyang H, Yuan H, Li J, Xie Z, et al. Site-specific Fat-1 knock-in enables significant decrease of n-6PUFAs/n-3PUFAs ratio in pigs. G3: Genes, Genomes, Genetics. 2018;**8**: 1747-1754. DOI: 10.1534/g3.118.200114

[99] Yan S, Tu Z, Liu Z, Fan N, Yang H, et al. A huntingtin knockin pig model recapitulates features of selective neurodegeneration in huntington's disease. Cell. 2018;**173**:989-1002.e13. DOI: 10.1016/j.cell.2018.03.005

[100] Zou Y, Li Z, Zou Y, Hao H, Li N, et al. An FBXO40 knockout generated by CRISPR/Cas9 causes muscle hypertrophy in pigs without detectable pathological effects. Biochemical and Biophysical Research Communications. 2018;**498**:940-945. DOI: 10.1016/j.bbrc.2018.03.085

[101] Yang H, Wang H, Shivalila CS, Cheng AW, Shi L, et al. One-step generation of mice carrying reporter and conditional alleles by CRISPR/Cas-mediated genome engineering. Cell. 2013;**154**:1370-1379. DOI: 10.1016/j.cell.2013.08.022

[102] Wang H, Yang H, Shivalila CS, Dawlaty MM, Cheng AW, et al. One-step generation of mice carrying

mutations in multiple genes by CRISPR/Cas-mediated genome engineering. Cell. 2013;**153**:910-918. DOI: 10.1016/j.cell.2013.04.025

[103] Fujii W, Kawasaki K, Sugiura K, Naito K. Efficient generation of large-scale genome-modified mice using gRNA and CAS9 endonuclease. Nucleic Acids Research. 2013;**41**:e187. DOI: 10.1093/nar/gkt772

[104] Shen B, Zhang J, Wu H, Wang J, Ma K, et al. Generation of gene-modified mice via Cas9/RNA-mediated gene targeting. Cell Research. 2013;**23**: 720-723. DOI: 10.1038/cr.2013.46

[105] Sato M, Koriyama M, Watanabe S, Ohtsuka M, Sakurai T, et al. Direct injection of CRISPR/Cas9-related mRNA into cytoplasm of parthenogenetically activated porcine oocytes causes frequent mosaicism for indel mutations. International Journal of Molecular Sciences. 2015;**16**:17838-17856. DOI: 10.3390/ijms160817838

[106] Sato M, Kosuke M, Koriyama M, Inada E, Saitoh I, et al. Timing of CRISPR/Cas9-related mRNA microinjection after activation as an important factor affecting genome editing efficiency in porcine oocytes. Theriogenology. 2018;**108**:29-38. DOI: 10.1016/j.theriogenology.2017.11.030

[107] Sung YH, Kim JM, Kim HT, Lee J, Jeon J, et al. Highly efficient gene knockout in mice and zebrafish with RNA-guided endonucleases. Genome Research. 2014;**24**:125-131. DOI: 10.1101/gr.163394.113

[108] Liang X, Potter J, Kumar S, Zou Y, Quintanilla R, et al. Rapid and highly efficient mammalian cell engineering via Cas9 protein transfection. Journal of Biotechnology. 2015;**208**:44-53. DOI: 10.1016/j.jbiotec.2015.04.024

[109] Jung CJ, Zhang J, Trenchard E, Lloyd KC, West DB, et al. Efficient gene targeting in mouse zygotes mediated by CRISPR/Cas9-protein. Transgenic Research. 2017;**26**:263-277. DOI: 10.1007/s11248-016-9998-5

[110] Aida T, Chiyo K, Usami T, Ishikubo H, Imahashi R, et al. Cloning-free CRISPR/Cas system facilitates functional cassette knock-in in mice. Genome Biology. 2015;**16**:87. DOI: 10.1186/s13059-015-0653-x

[111] Hashimoto M, Yamashita Y, Takemoto T. Electroporation of Cas9 protein/sgRNA into early pronuclear zygotes generates non-mosaic mutants in the mouse. Developmental Biology. 2016;**418**:1-9. DOI: 10.1016/j.ydbio.2016.07.017

[112] Tu Z, Yang W, Yan S, Yin A, Gao J, et al. Promoting Cas9 degradation reduces mosaic mutations in non-human primate embryos. Scientific Reports. 2017;**7**:42081. DOI: 10.1038/srep42081

[113] Huang Y, Tang X, Xie W, Zhou Y, Li D, et al. Vitamin C enhances *in vitro* and *in vivo* development of porcine somatic cell nuclear transfer embryos. Biochemical and Biophysical Research Communications. 2011;**411**:397-401. DOI: 10.1016/j.bbrc.2011.06.160

[114] Jeong YW, Park SW, Hossein MS. Anti-apoptotic and embryotrophic effects of a-tocopherol and L-ascorbic acid on porcine embryos derived from *in vitro* fertilisation and somatic cell nuclear transfer. Theriogenology. 2006;**66**:2104-2112. DOI: 10.1016/j.theriogenology.2006.06.007

[115] Liang S, Jin YX, Yuan B, Zhang JB, Kim NH. Melatonin enhances the developmental competence of porcine somatic cell nuclear transfer embryos by preventing DNA damage induced by oxidative stress. Scientific Reports. 2017;**7**:11114. DOI: 10.1038/s41598-017-11161-9

[116] Wang XX, Jin YZ, Zuo ZR, Liu ZG. Replacement of glutamine with alanyl-glutamine dipeptide enhances the developmental competence of porcine (sus scrofa) embryos produced by somatic cell nuclear transfer. Journal of Agricultural Biotechnology. 2017;**25**:110-115

[117] Himaki T, Yokomine TA, Sato M, Takao S, Miyoshi K, et al. Effects of trichostatin A on *in vitro* development and transgene function in somatic cell nuclear transfer embryos derived from transgenic Clawn miniature pig cells. Animal Science Journal. 2010;**81**:558-563. DOI: 10.1111/j.1740-0929.2010.00772.x

[118] Cong P, Zhu K, Ji Q, Zhao H, Chen Y. Effects of trichostatin A on histone acetylation and methylation characteristics in early porcine embryos after somatic cell nuclear transfer. Journal of Animal Science. 2013;**84**: 639-649. DOI: 10.1111/asj.12059

[119] Miyoshi K, Mori H, Mizobe Y, Akasaka E, Ozawa A, et al. Valproic acid enhances *in vitro* development and Oct-3/4 expression of miniature pig somatic cell nuclear transfer embryos. Cellular Reprogramming. 2010;**12**:67-74. DOI: 10.1089/cell.2009.0032

[120] Huang Y, Tang X, Xie W, Zhou Y, Li D, et al. Histone deacetylase inhibitor significantly improved the cloning efficiency of porcine somatic cell nuclear transfer embryos. Cellular Reprogramming. 2011;**13**:513-520. DOI: 10.1089/cell.2011.0032

[121] Miyoshi K, Maeda K, Akioka K, Sato M, Kawaguchi H, et al. Birth of cloned microminipigs derived from somatic cell nuclear transfer embryos that have been transiently treated with valproic acid. Cellular Reprogramming. 2016;**18**: 390-400. DOI: 10.1089/cell.2016.0025

[122] Zhao J, Ross JW, Hao Y, Spate LD, Walters EM, et al. Significant improvement in cloning efficiency of an inbred miniature pig by histone deacetylase inhibitor treatment after somatic cell nuclear transfer. Biology of Reproduction. 2009;**81**:525-530. DOI: 10.1095/biolreprod.109.077016

[123] Zhao J, Hao Y, Ross JW, Spate LD, Walters EM, et al. Histone deacetylase inhibitors improve *in vitro* and *in vivo* developmental competence of somatic cell nuclear transfer porcine embryos. Cellular Reprogramming. 2010;**12**:75-83. DOI: 10.1089/cell.2009.0038

[124] Zhang L, Huang Y, Wu Y, Si J, Huang Y, et al. Scriptaid upregulates expression of development-related genes, inhibits apoptosis, and improves the development of somatic cell nuclear transfer mini-pig embryos. Cellular Reprogramming. 2017;**19**:19-26. DOI: 10.1089/cell.2016.0033

[125] Jin JX, Li S, Gao QS, Hong Y, Jin L, et al. Significant improvement of pig cloning efficiency by treatment with LBH589 after somatic cell nuclear transfer. Theriogenology. 2013;**80**:630-635. DOI: 10.1016/j.theriogenology.2013.06.006

[126] Hou L, Ma F, Yang J, Riaz H, Wang Y, et al. Effects of histone deacetylase inhibitor oxamflatin on *in vitro* porcine somatic cell nuclear transfer embryos. Cellular Reprogramming. 2014;**16**:253-265. DOI: 10.1089/cell.2013.0058

[127] Jin JX, Kang JD, Li S, Jin L, Zhu HY, et al. PXD101 significantly improves nuclear reprogramming and the *in vitro* developmental competence of porcine SCNT embryos. Biochemical and Biophysical Research Communications. 2015;**456**:156-161. DOI: 10.1016/j.bbrc.2014.11.051

[128] Jin L, Guo Q, Zhu HY, Xing XX, Zhang GL, et al. Quisinostat treatment improves histone acetylation and developmental competence of

porcine somatic cell nuclear transfer embryos. Molecular Reproduction and Development. 2017;**84**:340-346. DOI: 10.1002/mrd.22787

[129] Jin L, Zhu HY, Guo Q, Li XC, Zhang YC, et al. Effect of histone acetylation modification with MGCD0103, a histone deacetylase inhibitor, on nuclear reprogramming and the developmental competence of porcine somatic cell nuclear transfer embryos. Theriogenology. 2017;**87**:298-305. DOI: 10.1016/j.theriogenology.2016.09.011

[130] Zhang Z, Zhai Y, Ma X, Zhang S, An X, et al. Down-regulation of H3K4me3 by MM-102 facilitates epigenetic reprogramming of porcine somatic cell nuclear transfer embryos. Cellular Physiology and Biochemistry. 2018;**45**:1529-1540. DOI: 10.1159/000487579

[131] Lin T, Lee JE, Oqani RK, Kim SY, Cho ES, et al. Tauroursodeoxycholic acid improves pre-implantation development of porcine SCNT embryo by endoplasmic reticulum stress inhibition. Reproductive Biology. 2016;**16**:269-278. DOI: 10.1016/j.repbio.2016.10.003

[132] Wang P, Li X, Cao L, Huang S, Li H, et al. MicroRNA-148a overexpression improves the early development of porcine somatic cell nuclear transfer embryos. PLoS ONE. 2017;**12**:e0180535. DOI: 10.1371/journal.pone.0180535

[133] Matoba S, Liu Y, Lu F, Iwabuchi KA, Shen L, et al. Embryonic development following somatic cell nuclear transfer impeded by persisting histone methylation. Cell. 2014;**159**:884-895. DOI: 10.1016/j.cell.2014.09.055

[134] Kaneko T, Sakuma T, Yamamoto T, Mashimo T. Simple knockout by electroporation of engineered endonucleases into intact rat embryos. Scientific Reports. 2014;**4**:6382. DOI: 10.1038/srep06382

[135] Hashimoto M, Takemoto T. Electroporation enables the efficient mRNA delivery into the mouse zygotes and facilitates CRISPR/Cas9-based genome editing. Scientific Reports. 2015;**5**:11315. DOI: 10.1038/srep11315

[136] Qin W, Dion SL, Kutny PM, Zhang Y, Cheng AW, et al. Efficient CRISPR/Cas9-mediated genome editing in mice by zygote electroporation of nuclease. Genetics. 2015;**200**:423-430. DOI: 10.1534/genetics.115.176594

[137] Wei J, Gaynor P, Cole S, Brophy B, Oback B, et al. Developing the laboratory conditions for bovine zygote-mediated genome editing by electroporation. In: Proceedings of the World Congress on Genetics Applied to Livestock Production. Volume Technologies—Gene Editing; 2018. p. 1118

[138] Miyoshi N, Horiuchi M, Inokuchi Y, Miyamoto Y, Miura N, et al. Novel microminipig model of atherosclerosis by fat and high cholesterol diet, established in Japan. In Vivo. 2010;**24**:671-680

[139] Ohtsuka M, Sato M, Miura H, Takabayashi S, Matsuyama M, et al. i-GONAD: A robust method for in situ germline genome engineering using CRISPR nucleases. Genome Biology. 2018;**19**:25. DOI: 10.1186/s13059-018-1400-x

[140] Sato M, Miyoshi M, Nakamura S, Ohtsuka M, Sakurai T, et al. Efficient generation of somatic cell nuclear transfer-competent porcine cells with mutated alleles at multiple target loci by using CRISPR/Cas9 combined with targeted toxin-based selection system. International Journal of Molecular Sciences. 2017;**18**:2610. DOI: 10.3390/ijms18122610

[141] Sakurai T, Watanabe S, Kamiyoshi A, Sato M, Shindo T. A single blastocyst assay optimized for detecting CRISPR/Cas9 system-induced indel mutations in

mice. BMC Biotechnology. 2014;**14**:69. DOI: 10.1186/1472-6750-14-69

[142] Akasaka E, Ozawa A, Mori H, Mizobe Y, Yoshida M, et al. Whole-genome amplification-based GenomiPhi for multiple genomic analysis of individual early porcine embryos. Theriogenology. 2011;**75**:1543-1549. DOI: 10.1016/j.theriogenology.2010.12.018

[143] Fu Y, Foden JA, Khayter C, Maeder ML, Reyon D, et al. High-frequency off-target mutagenesis induced by CRISPR-Cas nucleases in human cells. Nature Biotechnology. 2013;**31**:822-826. DOI: 10.1038/nbt.2623

[144] Ran FA, Hsu PD, Lin CY, Gootenberg JS, Konermann S, et al. Double nicking by RNA-guided CRISPR Cas9 for enhanced genome editing specificity. Cell. 2013;**154**:1380-1389. DOI: 10.1016/j.cell.2013.08.021

[145] Kim S, Kim D, Cho SW, Kim J, Kim JS. Highly efficient RNA-guided genome editing in human cells via delivery of purified Cas9 ribonucleoproteins. Genome Research. 2014;**24**:1012-1019. DOI: 10.1101/gr.171322.113

[146] Guilinger JP, Thompson DB, Liu DR. Fusion of catalytically inactive Cas9 to FokI nuclease improves the specificity of genome modification. Nature Biotechnology. 2014;**32**:577-582. DOI: 10.1038/nbt.2909

[147] Zetsche B, Gootenberg JS, Abudayyeh OO, Slaymaker IM, Makarova KS, et al. Cpf1 is a single RNA-guided endonuclease of a class 2 CRISPR-Cas system. Cell. 2015;**163**: 759-771. DOI: 10.1016/j.cell.2015.09.038

[148] Slaymaker IM, Gao L, Zetsche B, Scott DA, Yan WX, et al. Rationally engineered Cas9 nucleases with improved specificity. Science. 2016;**351**:84-88. DOI: 10.1126/science.aad5227

[149] Kleinstiver BP, Pattanayak V, Prew MS, Tsai SQ, Nguyen NT, et al. High-fidelity CRISPR-Cas9 nucleases with no detectable genome-wide off-target effects. Nature. 2016;**529**: 490-495. DOI: 10.1038/nature16526

[150] Nishida K, Arazoe T, Yachie N, Banno S, Kakimoto M, et al. Targeted nucleotide editing using hybrid prokaryotic and vertebrate adaptive immune systems. Science. 2016;353:pii: aaf8729. DOI:10.1126/science.aaf8729

[151] Abudayyeh OO, Gootenberg JS, Essletzbichler P, Han S, Joung J, et al. RNA targeting with CRISPR-Cas13. Nature. 2017;**550**:280-284. DOI: 10.1038/nature24049

[152] Cong L, Ran FA, Cox D, Lin S, Barretto R, et al. Multiplex genome engineering using CRISPR/Cas systems. Science. 2013;**339**:819-823. DOI: 10.1126/science.1231143

[153] Mali P, Yang L, Esvelt KM, Aach J, Guell M, et al. RNA-guided human genome engineering via Cas9. Science. 2013;**339**:823-826. DOI: 10.1126/science.1232033

[154] Sakurai T, Kamiyoshi A, Kawate H, Mori C, Watanabe S, et al. A non-inheritable maternal Cas9-based multiple-gene editing system in mice. Scientific Reports. 2016;**6**:20011. DOI: 10.1038/srep20011

[155] Mao Z, Bozzella M, Seluanov A, Gorbunova V. Comparison of nonhomologous end joining and homologous recombination in human cells. DNA Repair (Amst). 2008;**7**: 1765-1771. DOI: 10.1016/j.dnarep.2008.06.018

[156] Maruyama T, Dougan SK, Truttmann MC, Bilate AM, Ingram JR, et al. Increasing the efficiency of precise genome editing with CRISPR-Cas9 by inhibition of nonhomologous

end joining. Nature Biotechnology. 2015;**33**:538-542. DOI: 10.1038/nbt.3190

[157] Chu VT, Weber T, Wefers B, Wurst W, Sander S, et al. Increasing the efficiency of homology-directed repair for CRISPR-Cas9-induced precise gene editing in mammalian cells. Nature Biotechnology. 2015;**33**:543-548. DOI: 10.1038/nbt.3198

[158] Song J, Yang D, Xu J, Zhu T, Chen YE, et al. RS-1 enhances CRISPR/Cas9- and TALEN-mediated knock-in efficiency. Nature Communications. 2016;**7**:10548. DOI: 10.1038/ncomms10548

[159] Gerlach M, Kraft T, Brenner B, Petersen B, Niemann H, et al. Efficient knock-in of a point mutation in porcine fibroblasts using the CRISPR/Cas9-GMNN fusion gene. Genes. 2018;**9**:296. DOI: 10.3390/genes9060296

[160] Li G, Zhang X, Zhong C, Mo J, Quan R, et al. Small molecules enhance CRISPR/Cas9-mediated homology-directed genome editing in primary cells. Scientific Reports. 2017;**7**:8943. DOI: 10.1038/s41598-017-09306-x

[161] Platt RJ, Chen S, Zhou Y, Yim MJ, Swiech L, et al. CRISPR-Cas9 knockin mice for genome editing and cancer modeling. Cell. 2014;**159**:440-455. DOI: 10.1016/j.cell.2014.09.014

[162] Cebrian-Serrano A, Zha S, Hanssen L, Biggs D, Preece C, et al. Maternal supply of Cas9 to zygotes facilitates the efficient generation of site-specific mutant mouse models. PLoS ONE. 2017;**12**:e0169887. DOI: 10.1371/journal.pone.0169887

[163] Wang K, Jin Q, Ruan D, Yang Y, Liu Q, et al. Cre-dependent Cas9-expressing pigs enable efficient *in vivo* genome editing. Genome Research. 2017;**27**:2061-2071. DOI: 10.1101/gr.222521.117

Section 2

Other Species

Chapter 6

A Review of the Macroscopic, Microscopic, and Ultramicroscopic Characteristics of Some Key Oocyte Developmental Processes in Fish Species

Mônica Cassel

Abstract

Studies involving the reproductive biology of fish have several possibilities of approach, such as the understanding of gonadal development, oocyte development, and the reproductive cycle of the species. In addition, analyses of gonadal morphology can be made at macro-, micro-, and ultramicroscopic levels. This knowledge helps to define factors that determine the different stages of gonadal development, as well as the "triggers" that initiate the reproductive process. In females, the growth and maturation of the ovarian follicles depend on a carefully elaborated communication between the follicular cells and the oocyte and a precisely organized contractile system. Changes in these systems appear to be related to apoptotic cells. This extensive remodeling of gonadal tissue, due to cell proliferation and differentiation, promotes also changes in the extracellular matrix. With this in mind, we provide herein a complementary and in-depth information on cell-cell and cell-matrix interactions related to the process of oocyte development in fish species. This information, together with the existing structural and ultrastructural descriptions of ovaries of different species, will enable a better understanding of the reproductive processes for the group of fish.

Keywords: fish species, reproductive biology, gonadal and oocyte development, cell-cell interactions, cell-matrix interactions

1. Introduction

The knowledge on the reproductive characteristics of fish is fundamental to understand the adaptations developed to maximize the reproductive success in a given environment, considering the life history aspects of each species [1]. Studies involving the reproductive biology of fish have several possibilities of approach, such as the understanding of gonadal development and the reproductive cycle of the species. Analyses of gonadal morphology are important for the understanding of the biology of the species and have been widely applied in

Teleostei, as in recent studies on spermatogenesis [2–5], folliculogenesis [6–8], reproductive cycle [8–12], and fecundity [13].

Studies have been carried out to describe and classify the stages of gonadal development and reproductive stages of fish in the Neotropical region. One of the most classic and used bibliographic sources has been Vazzoler [14]. However, other proposals for description have already been made by Grier and Taylor [15], Grier [16], and Lo Nostro et al. [17], which detail the continuity and discontinuity of the germinal epithelium and the cell types present in the gonads. Recently, Brown-Peterson et al. [18] developed a simpler terminology to facilitate the communication and comparison of studies on the reproductive biology of fish. Still in order to make the nomenclature more comprehensive, the stages of oocyte development were simplified by Quagio-Grassiotto et al. [19], and the development of stages of atresia, which are characterized as involutive processes, follows according to Miranda et al. [20].

Gonadal development can be analyzed macroscopically, and changes in shape, size, color, and texture of the gonads have been used as parameters for the classification of maturation status in many studies of ecology and reproductive dynamics[14, 21]. However, the most used analysis has been of the microscopic characters, since it allows a more detailed and precise description of the transitions and morphological and structural transformations that happen during gonadal development [8, 22, 23]. Thus, regarding the microscopic aspects of the gonad, it is verified that [24]:

- Spermatogenesis shows stages of development that include spermatogonia, spermatocytes, spermatids, and spermatozoa.

- Oogenesis usually shows the following progression: oogonia, primary growth oocytes, a previtellogenic stage in which oocytes grow larger and often have cortical alveolar vesicles, an extensive vitellogenic phase, oocyte maturation, and ovulation.

The oocyte development in a mature egg is a complex process modulated by numerous environmental and endocrine factors [25], and understanding the morphological characteristics of oocytes is important to interpret the dynamics of oogenesis [26]. Among the oocyte processes, folliculogenesis results in the removal of the primary oocyte from oogonium nests and consequent formation of ovarian follicles [27]. Descriptions for the germinal epithelium made by Grier [28] conceptualized "follicular complex" as the functional unit of the ovary. This complex is formed by two compartments separated by a basement membrane. One compartment is the follicle, which consists of the oocyte surrounded by follicular cells and originated from the germinal epithelium. The second compartment is the theca, made up of undifferentiated ovarian stromal cells.

In the previtellogenic oocyte phase, multiple nucleoli are observed, as described by Grier et al. [29]. These oocytes are also called perinucleolar oocytes, when the nucleoli migrate to the nuclear periphery. There is also the formation of the zona pellucida, a complex structure consisting generally of two layers crossed by pores or channels containing the oocyte microvilli and/or follicular cell extensions. The zona pellucida reflects adaptations to different ecological conditions in which the eggs develop [30], whose inner layer protects the egg from mechanical damage and whose outer layer protects it from microorganisms.

Another cell characteristic that is used to describe the stages of oocyte development is the presence of nüages, Balbiani corpuscles, and cortical alveoli. The nüages are originated by the transfer from the nucleus to the cytoplasm of large amounts of heterogeneous and ribosomal RNA synthesized [31] and associated with proteins. Balbiani corpuscles or yolk nuclei, described by Hubbard [32], were recognized as clusters of organelles located near the nucleus, which proliferate intensely and spread throughout the cytoplasm. And, the cortical alveoli, as observed by Grier et al. [29], are vesicles filled with glycoproteins, formed by depressions of the oocyte membrane that become progressively larger, marking the final stage of primary or previtellogenic growth.

The described changes are followed by an expressive growth of the oocyte during vitellogenesis, in which the oocyte accumulates the nutritive reserves necessary for the development of the embryo. The oocyte also accumulates RNA and completes the differentiation of its cellular and noncellular envelopes. During this time, the oocyte interrupts the meiosis at the end of the prophase and in the diplotene stage. Maturation processes are characterized by the reduction or halting of endocytosis, resumption of meiosis, breakdown of the germinal vesicle, formation of a monolayer of cortical alveoli under the plasma oocyte membrane, and dissolution of yolk platelets; pelagic oocytes still undergo hydration [6].

The understanding of cellular modifications is used to describe the reproductive cycle. This allows the recognition of the reproduction period and the gonadal morphological changes that occur. Descriptions of the reproductive cycle were initially elaborated by Yamamoto [33] and Agostinho et al. [34, 35], revalidated by Vazzoler [14], and later used by many authors. Next, Nuñez and Duponchelle [10] defined five stages of ovarian development with greater cellular detail and other four stages of testicular development based on macro- and microscopic characteristics. The last descriptions made by Lowerre-Barbieri et al. [24] and Quagio-Grassiotto et al. [19] on oocyte development, coupled with the stages of the reproductive cycle described by Brown-Peterson et al. [18], brought a proposal to homogenize the terms used and that has been applied in more recent studies. Research on the reproductive cycle of a given species helps to define determinant phases of gonadal development, as well as the "triggers" that initiate the process of cell proliferation and differentiation in the formation of gametes [14, 36–38].

2. Important cellular morphological modifications during the oocyte development process

2.1 Cellular junctions and your distribution throughout the oocyte development

The growth and maturation of the ovarian follicles depend on carefully crafted communication between the somatic cells of the follicle and the oocyte. This association between somatic cell and germ cell in the ovaries of various vertebrate and invertebrate species is established through intercellular junctions [39–43]. In vertebrate ovarian follicles, direct cytoplasmic connections between the oocyte and follicular cells of the granulosa layer associated with it are established early in the oocyte development. In fish, amphibians, and mammals, these cytoplasmic connections are established at the points of contact between the oocyte microvilli and follicular cells or between follicular cell microvilli and oocyte, via specialized membrane junctions known as GAP junctions [44–47].

GAP junctions are intermembrane channel aggregates between adjacent cells composed by connexin proteins [48]. These junctions are considered homologous when they connect follicular cells to follicular cells and heterologous when they connect follicular cells to the oocyte [49]. Recent observations suggest that the functional coupling of GAP junctions, especially homologous ones, is necessary for the occurrence of the oocyte maturation process [50]. A possible role for the heterologous GAP junctions is the transfer of cAMP (PKA activator) from the follicular cells to the oocyte in order to induce the production or activity of membrane receptors for the maturation-inducing hormone, or MIH [50], indirectly participating in the oocyte maturation process. GAP junctions may also be involved in specifying the pattern of polarity in the oocytes of various animal groups, so this junctional route can be used to pass intercellular signals from follicular cells to the oocyte to determine oocyte symmetry [51].

As previously reported, the fish oocyte is enveloped by the zona pellucida (microvillus area), by the follicular cells and by the basement membrane. Thus, from a morphological and functional point of view, it is important to know if there are any tight junctions between adjacent follicular cells, since these joints promote barriers for the passage of fluids through the extracellular space between adjacent cell membranes and maintain tissue and cell integrity [45, 52–54]. The main components of the intercellular junctions are the tight junctions [55, 56], which are composed of different transmembrane proteins that promote a homophilic interaction. The cytoplasmic domain of the transmembrane adhesion molecules connects the binding proteins which, in turn, anchor the cytoskeletal adhesion complex. Of these molecules, occludins and claudins are the most extensively studied. Although occludin is a highly conserved molecule, claudins comprise a family of more than 20 different proteins, some of which are expressed in a tissue-specific manner [57–59].

As claudins, cadherins are a transmembrane superfamily of proteins that contain several homologous members, exhibiting tissue diversity and distinct binding specificities [60–62], with a highly conserved cytoplasmic domain [63, 64]. These molecules mediate cell-cell contact at adhesion junctions also anchored in the cytoskeleton, thus playing an important role in the separation, positioning and control of cell movements, and in morphogenesis [65–67]. In a study with *Danio rerio*, E-cadherin homologous proteins were identified, and their synthesis and storage during oogenesis were verified [62]. Also, the establishment of heterotypic junctions linking the oocyte to follicular cells throughout folliculogenesis and cooperating in the determination of follicle architecture was observed [62]. When oocytes progress in vitellogenesis, the localization of adhesion proteins in the oocyte becomes restricted to a more specific pattern, which reflects the points of contact between the oocyte and the follicle cells and their adjustment to changes in the oocyte cytoskeleton throughout this phase [62].

2.2 Distribution and structuration of the cytoskeleton throughout the oocyte development

All intracytoplasmic and cortical events in oocytes involve a precisely organized and collaborative contractile system and a stable support matrix [68]. The cytoskeleton of the oocytes and embryos is implicated in key developmental events, such as creation and maintenance of axial polarity, cytoplasmic reorganization, cell division, change of surface architecture, morphogenetic motions, and internal arrangement of organelles [69]. It seems very likely that cytoskeletal structures are responsible for spatial distribution of yolk, cortical and pigment granules, lipid droplets, or mitochondria [68, 70]. Thus, the spatial organization of cytoskeletal filaments may be important for the preservation of oocyte viability [71].

Among the different proteins expressed in the cytoskeleton, the intermediate filament proteins are exceptionally complex [72, 73], especially in the class of cytokeratins. This is a class of proteins typical and specifically induced in cells compromised for epithelial differentiation [72, 74, 75], and their identification in oocytes and eggs presents an interesting contrast when comparing to other cytoskeletal proteins in germ cells. Cytokeratins are not synthesized in previtellogenic oocytes but are expressed and accumulated in the vitellogenic stage. These filament proteins are first detectable in the cortex of oocytes in later stages of previtellogenesis; at the beginning of vitellogenesis, they are distributed primarily in the region closest to the nucleus and appear to become cortical again in mature oocytes [76]. Intermediate filaments of cytokeratin contribute to the complex structure of the oocyte and egg cortex, which is also rich in other cytoskeletal filaments such as actin filaments and microtubules [68, 77–79].

The microtubule matrix seems to be a very important component in the immature oocyte cortex in fish. The function of the cortical matrix of microtubules in oocytes remains undetermined but may be related to the mechanical stiffness that has been attributed to the cortex [80]. Even the basic mechanism of germinal vesicle migration and its mechanical anchoring in the region of the animal pole occur from the depolarization of the microtubules, leading to a consequent change in the position of the germinal vesicle [80, 81].

Evident changes occur in the distribution and localization of tubulin-containing structures in growing oocytes. In previtellogenic oocytes, a great amount of tubulin is concentrated in the Balbiani corpuscle [82–85]. During vitellogenesis, mitochondria are displaced from the Balbiani corpuscle to the surface of the cell, while others remain around the nucleus [82, 86], and this movement seems to be related to the reorganization of tubulin [87]. With the disintegration of the Balbiani corpuscle, due to the anterior displacement of membranous organelles, the released space is gradually filled with yolk, i.e., the yolk granules are in a tubulin-positive region. As vitellogenesis progresses, rearrangement of cell growth and its contents occurs with the movement of endosomes to transport yolk through the microtubules [87].

The proper organization and assembly of the cytoskeleton microtubule is an integral phenomenon, which is related to the expression of cellular asymmetry. Particularly in oocytes, the microtubules exhibit a unique paradigm as forming an eccentric meiotic spindle which, consequently, gives rise to asymmetric cytokinesis to form the first and second polar bodies. Its existence and function are dynamically regulated throughout the process of cell division, particularly during the S and M phases of the cell cycle [88].

Another element that contributes to the oocyte asymmetry is the actin cytoskeleton. In oocytes, the actin filaments are not randomly distributed within the cell [89]. In germ cells, as in many other cells, two types of actin are present: filamentous (F-actin) and non-filamentous (G-actin) actins [90]. Actin polymerization-depolymerization process is essential for the translocation of many organelles, as mitochondria [91], Golgi system [92], and cortical granules [93, 94], as well as for the regulation of ion channel activity [95]. In addition, a certain proportion of F-actin and G-actin is required for the normal course of meiotic and mitotic divisions [96].

In many cells, a significant part of these filaments is in the area of the cellular cortex, so it has been proposed that they take part in the transduction of transmembrane information signals, including hormonal signaling [97, 98]. Still in the oocyte cortex, the cortex-specific F-actin layer is peculiarly absent in the space between the germinal vesicle and the plasma membrane at the animal pole. In fact, it is through this "corridor" that the two polar bodies are extruded in the posterior phase of meiosis [99, 100].

The formation of actin bundles in the oocyte cortex is one of the first morphological markers of induction to maturation [99]. The role of actin microfilaments in oocyte maturation seems to be related to the translocation of the endoplasmic reticulum structures to the germinal vesicle area and to the coordination of the cortical granules in the plasma membrane zone [93, 101]. Even during follicular atresia, the actin cytoskeleton undergoes changes associated with the yolk degradation, while it remains preserved in follicular cells. Thus, maintenance of the actin cytoskeleton may be a sign of survival for follicular cells during early and/or advanced atresia processes [102]. Cytoskeleton changes have been extensively reported in apoptotic cells, among which changes in cell shape and anchorage are dependent on the reorganization of actin filaments and focal adhesion contacts [103].

3. Morphological characteristics related to ovarian reorganization

3.1 Processes of atresia and cellular proliferation

Atresia is a degenerative process by which the ovarian follicles lose their integrity and are eliminated [104]. It is a common process in vertebrate ovaries under natural and/or experimental conditions [105] and can be induced by a series of exogenous and endogenous factors [106–109]. Oocyte degeneration, or follicular atresia, is a process that may occur before spawning, in oocytes that have not reached maturity and thereafter in oocytes that are no longer ovulated [110, 111]. In fish, atresia is involved in normal ovary growth [112, 113] and postovulatory regression [114–116], especially in females that are not able to perform maturation or ovulation after the vitellogenesis process [117].

Fish, in general, exhibits a reproductive periodicity, and, therefore, oocytes at various stages of development may be resorbed with the resultant formation of an atretic body. Considering the foregoing, Rajalakshmi [118] made a classification of the atretic processes taking into account the following stages: (1) "immature oocyte atresia" begins with the distortion of the cell shape, followed by loss of cytoplasmic homogeneity and reabsorption of the structure (in this type of atresia, the follicular cells do not exhibit any activity so the reabsorption of oocytes without yolk seems to be a relatively simple process); (2) "mature oocyte atresia" begins with the loss of the soft outline of the zona pellucida and dissociation of the follicular cells, which will then present phagocytic characteristic (i.e., enzymatic activity of acid phosphatase that will liquefy the yolk), followed by a slow dissolution of the zona pellucida and culminating in total resorption of the follicle; (3) "postovulatory complex atresia" begins with the distortion of the follicular cell shape, followed by loss of cell boundaries and formation of a syncytial structure, and finally the follicle shrink, with consequent degenerative changes.

The morphological characteristics of the atretic bodies and their stages of involution, independent of cellular development stage, were summarized in the study of Miranda et al. [20], as (1) initial atresia, with the disintegration of the oocyte nucleus, fragmentation of the zona pellucida, and follicular cell hypertrophy; (2) intermediate atresia, with follicular cells presenting phagocytic characteristics and ingesting the yolk; (3) advanced atresia, with numerous myelinic figures in the cytoplasm of follicular cells; and (4) final atresia, with the reduction in the number of follicular and theca cells and presence of granules of lipofuscin and granulocytes near the atretic follicle. With the current emergence of the theme of cell death pathways, studies about ovarian involutive processes in fish were brought to the spotlight again with new descriptions being made [102, 108, 116, 119–124] that add and/or corroborate those morphological characteristics already proposed by Miranda et al. [20].

In fish, mammals and, presumably, other vertebrates, the molecular mechanism responsible for ovarian follicular atresia is cell death by apoptosis [102, 124, 125]. Apoptosis, or programmed cell death, is a physiological process controlled by various hormones and growth factors. This is an evolutionarily conserved process, involved in remodeling, differentiation, and tissue degeneration in a variety of cell types [125]. It is characterized by biochemical and morphological changes such as chromatin condensation, DNA fragmentation, and the formation of apoptotic bodies [126]. The main effector proteins in apoptosis are the caspases, a family of highly conserved cysteine proteases [127, 128]. Among the caspases, caspase-3 is the major effector one, including in the ovarian tissue in which it is expressed in the follicular cells of atretic follicles of fish and mammals [102, 124, 129].

In addition to apoptosis, Thomé et al. [130] presented a new route to cell death—the autophagy. This route differs from apoptosis by the purpose of the processes:

apoptosis is the programmed cell death, and autophagy is a stress adaptation to prevent cell death. The functional relationship between apoptosis and autophagy is complex. In some cases, autophagy is a form of adaptation to suppress apoptosis, whereas, in other cases, autophagy constitutes an alternative pathway of cellular elimination called autophagic or type II cell death [131–133]. It has been understood that apoptosis is the main mechanism involved in the involution of postovulatory follicles [116, 121], while autophagy contributes to the regression of atretic follicles [20, 130]. Even though the limits and interrelationships between these two processes have not yet been well established, recent studies have shown that there may be a crosstalk between autophagy and apoptosis pathways in the ovarian involution processes. A fine balance between the signs for survival and cell death appears to be essential for determining the fate of follicular cells, particularly in follicular atresia [102, 124].

During follicular development, a low rate of follicular cell apoptosis can be considered as a physiological event for the control of the appropriate number of cells and elimination of the undesirable ones [134]. However, high apoptosis values can be observed under unfavorable conditions, compromising follicular viability [135]. Thus, organic homeostasis is dependent on the balance between cell proliferation, differentiation, and death, so populations of rapidly proliferating cells usually have high rates of cell death by apoptosis [125, 136].

The mechanism of cell proliferation is a highly regulated process that seems to be essential for the maintenance of ovarian homeostasis [137], and yet the hormonal mechanism controlling oocyte proliferation and recruitment of oocytes is not understood completely for any vertebrate [6]. In contrast to mammals, oogonia continue to proliferate in adult female fish [138], thus renewing stocks of young oocytes and follicles [139, 140]. The pre-follicular and follicular cells begin to proliferate when in the folliculogenesis phase, to support the oocyte growth [19]. However, ovarian mitosis in fish is usually observed at the end of each reproductive cycle [137], when ovarian tissues are reorganized [141, 142]. Throughout ovigerous lamellae in adult females, germ cell proliferation and the formation of germline cysts result in extensions of the germinal epithelium that are segregated from the connective tissue by a basement membrane [19]. These extensions of the germinal epithelium are known as oogonium nests [28, 143] and mark the beginning of the reproductive cycle again.

3.2 Extracellular matrix and its changes through the reproductive cycle

During the reproductive cycle, ovarian tissue is constantly remodeled, with extensive cell proliferation and differentiation, as well as extracellular matrix changes from early follicular development to tissue involution after ovulation [144]. Among the processes and factors involved in tissue remodeling are apoptosis, changes in hormone levels, and degradation of the extracellular matrix in contact with cells [134].

The extracellular matrix is an insoluble network of several structural and functional macromolecules found in connective tissues and basement membranes [145]. It is both a barrier that separates the organism into tissue compartments and a substrate for cell adhesion [146]. In addition to these structural functions, the extracellular matrix is an essential regulator of cellular physiology, predominantly in cell survival, cell cycle, cell migration, and morphogenesis [147].

A coordinated interaction of signals is necessary to regulate the proliferation, differentiation, adhesion, and migration of specific cell types for the development and organization of structural tissues [148]. During the normal development of an organ or in pathological modifications, the matrix undergoes intense changes in its composition. This process, called matrix remodeling, is involved in many physiological processes, such as activation of immune cells [149], wound healing [150, 151], embryogenesis [152, 153], or reproductive cycle [154].

The extracellular matrix-cell interactions influence gene regulation, cytoskeletal structure, differentiation, and many aspects of cell growth [155]. Changes in the expression of components that make up the extracellular matrix accompany follicular growth, ovulation, and involution of postovulatory follicles, which in its turn may influence follicular maturation, cell survival, and steroidogenesis [134, 156, 157]. Studies with mammals demonstrate that gonadal support cells synthesize a variety of components comprising the extracellular matrix and the basement membrane, such as collagen, laminin, keratin, fibronectin, lectin, and fibril chains [158, 159].

The balance between the degradation and regeneration of the extracellular matrix in ovarian tissues is maintained, in part, by the action of extracellular proteolytic enzymes that are secreted by the local cells. Most of these enzymes are matrix metalloproteinases (MMPs), which depend on the Ca^{+2} or Zn^{+2} binding to their activity [160]. During oogenesis, great changes in the extracellular environment of the ovary were largely attributed to the action of MMPs [144]. MMPs play an important role in the ovulation process in different groups of vertebrates, acting on follicular rupture, basement membrane fragmentation, and follicular connective fibers [144, 161, 162].

The integrity of the basement membrane is also evidenced by the continuous marking of laminin-β2 and type IV collagen, which allows the development of ovarian follicles [159, 163]. On the other hand, the discontinuous labeling of laminin-β2 and type IV collagen in the basal membrane of postovulatory follicles indicates that basement membrane degradation occurs due to the breakdown of these major components [134]. The loss of the basement membrane integrity may contribute to the increase of follicular cell apoptosis, suggesting its influence on the survival of postovulatory follicle cells [116].

Fibronectin and laminin have been shown to be extracellular matrix proteins synthesized by follicular cells [164, 165]. The presence of fibronectin on the surface of postovulatory follicle cells is due to the need of interaction between their domains with type IV collagen and cell surface integrin, and it is important for the maintenance of cell adhesion in the extracellular matrix [159]. According to Iwahashi et al. [166], the type IV collagen detected in the connective tissue among theca cells may be involved in the organization of extracellular fibronectin. This interaction between type IV collagen and fibronectin may act on cell migration that occurs during the late remodeling of postovulatory follicles [134].

Thus, the structure and composition of the extracellular matrix play an important role during follicular development and post-spawning involution in teleost fish. The basement membrane integrity is important for follicular cell survival, and the loss of integrity contributes to increased follicular apoptosis. In addition, MMP-9 may be involved in the final oocyte maturation and regression of postovulatory follicles [134]. Therefore, it follows that different combinations and proportions in the assembly of extracellular matrix components, together with the presentation of a large variety of proteoglycans at various times during the development and maturation of the gonads, can orchestrate distinct gene expression programs and culminate in more diverse tissue variations and adaptations [148].

4. Conclusions

Studies in gametogenesis help to understand the ecological, adaptive, and evolutionary relationships in the groups of species, especially when the oocyte structures are analyzed in an ultrastructural level. This is even more important when we consider that there are few fish species that present descriptions with adequate morphological and/or functional detail. Most of the studies do not evaluate the reproductive characteristics with the necessary histological and ultrastructural details, which can lead to incomplete interpretations of the reproductive characteristics of the species. Likewise, studies involving organelles and their distribution throughout the reproductive cycle and cellular development in fish species are punctual or restricted to a developmental stage. The understanding of these processes is then due to the sum of several studies at different stages of development, but they do not necessarily represent the same environmental, behavioral, and population pressures that are being addressed to the individuals of a given species. Thus, the continuous study of these variables throughout the reproductive cycle of key species may allow more real parameters on the dynamics of the intracellular structures in germ cells and follicular cells, as well as the extracellular matrix. All of the above is even more relevant when applied to such a diverse group, as fish, that have great ecological, social, and economic importance.

Acknowledgements

I would like to thank all those who did or are part of the laboratories where I conducted my undergraduate and graduate studies and who culminated in the improvement of the knowledge reproduced here. I thank Dr. Adelina Ferreira, Dr. Mahmoud Mehanna, and Dr. Débora Fabiane Neves da Silva, advisors and colleagues at the Morphology and Morphometry Laboratory of the Federal University of Mato Grosso (UFMT), for the first steps taken in the area of Animal Reproduction. I would also like to thank Dr. Maria Inês Borella, Dr. Chayrra Chehade Gomes, Dr. Gisele Cristiane de Melo Dias, Dr. Lázaro Wender Oliveira de Jesus, MSc Giovana de Souza Branco, MSc Marília de Paiva Camargo, and laboratory technician Cruz Alberto Mendoza Rigonatti of the Laboratory of Fish Endocrinology, University of São Paulo, for the support during the doctorate and for all the knowledge obtained in that period. Lastly, I would like to thank the FAPEMAT, CAPES, and FAPESP funding agencies for the financial support provided during my academic trajectory, which culminated in the formulation of this chapter.

Conflict of interest

The author declares that there is no conflict of interest regarding the publication of this chapter.

Author details

Mônica Cassel
Mato Grosso Federal Institute of Education, Science and Technology—Campus Alta Floresta, Alta Floresta, MT, Brazil

*Address all correspondence to: cassel.mcp@gmail.com

References

[1] Mazzoni R, Mendonça RS, Caramaschi EP. Reproductive biology of *Astyanax janeiroensis* (Osteichthyes, Characidae) from the Ubatiba River, Maricá, RJ, Brazil. Brazilian Journal of Biology. 2005;**65**(4):643-649. DOI: 10.1590/S1519-69842005000400012

[2] Nóbrega RH, Batlouni SR, França LR. An overview of functional and stereological evaluation of spermatogenesis and germ cell transplantation in fish. Fish Physiology and Biochemistry. 2008;**35**(1):197-206. DOI: 10.1007/s10695-008-9252-z

[3] Schulz RW, França LR, Lareyre JJ, Legac F, Chiarini-Garcia H, Nóbrega RH, et al. Spermatogenesis in fish. General and Comparative Endocrinology. 2010;**165**(3):390-411. DOI: 10.1016/j.ygcen.2009.02.013

[4] Costa FG, Adolfi MC, Gomes CC, Jesus LWO, Batlouni SR, Borella MI. Tests of *Astyanax altiparanae*:The Sertoli cell functions in a semicystic spermatogenesis. Micron. 2014;**61**:20-27. DOI: 10.1016/j.micron.2014.02.004

[5] Camargo MP, Cassel M, Jesus LWO, Nóbrega RH, Borella MI. Characterization of undifferentiated spermatogonia and the spermatogonial niche in the lambari fish *Astyanax altiparanae*. Theriogenology. 2017;**96**:97-102. DOI: 10.1016/j.theriogenology.2017.03.027

[6] Lubzens E, Young G, Bobe J, Cerdà J. Oogenesis in teleosts: How fish eggs are formed. General and Comparative Endocrinology. 2010;**165**(3):367-389. DOI: 10.1016/j.ygcen.2009.05.022

[7] Martins YS, Moura DF, Santos GB, Rizzo E, Bazzoli N. Comparative folliculogenesis and spermatogenesis of four teleost fish from a reservoir in south-eastern Brazil. Acta Zoologica. 2010;**91**(4):466-473. DOI: 10.1111/j.1463-6395.2009.00437.x

[8] Cassel M, Chehade C, Branco GS, Canepelle D, Romagosa E, Borella MI. Ovarian development and the reproductive profile of *Astyanax altiparanae* (Teleostei, Characidae) over one year: Applications in fish farming. Theriogenology. 2017;**98**:1-15. DOI: 10.1016/j.theriogenology.2017.04.044

[9] Carvalho PA, Paschoalini AL, Santos GB, Rizzo E, Bazzoli N. Reproductive biology of *Astyanax fasciatus* (Pisces: Characiformes) in a reservoir in southeastern Brazil. Journal of Applied Ichthyology. 2009;**25**(3):306-313. DOI: 10.1111/j.1439-0426.2009.01238.x

[10] Nuñez K, Duponchelle F. Towards a universal scale to assess sexual maturation and related life history traits in oviparous teleost fishes. Fish Physiology and Biochemistry. 2009;**35**(1):167-180. DOI: 10.1007/s10695-008-9241-2

[11] Casali RCV, Vono V, Godinho HP, Luz RK, Bazzoli N. Passage and reproductive activity of fishes in the Igarapava fish ladder, Grande River, southeastern Brazil. River Research and Applications. 2010;**26**(2):157-165. DOI: 10.1002/rra.1242

[12] Chehade C, Cassel M, Borella MI. Induced reproduction in a migratory teleost species by water level drawdown. Neotropical Ichthyology. 2015;**13**(1):205-212. DOI: 10.1590/1982-0224-20140028

[13] Normando FT, Arantes FP, Luz RK, Thomé RG, Rizzo E, Sato Y, et al. Reproduction and fecundity of tucunaré, *Cichla kelberi* (Perciformes: Cichlidae), an exotic species in Três Marias reservoir, south eastern Brazil. Journal of Applied Ichthyology. 2009;**25**(3):299-305. DOI: 10.1111/j.1439-0426.2008.01174.x

[14] Vazzoler AEAM. Biologia da reprodução de peixes teleósteos: teoria e prática. Maringá: Eduem; 1996. 169 p

[15] Grier HJ, Taylor RG. Testicular maturation and regression in the common snook. Journal of Fish Biology. 1998;**53**(3):521-542. DOI: 10.1111/j.1095-8649.1998.tb00999.x

[16] Grier HJ. The germinal epithelium: Its dual role in establishing male reproductive classes and understanding the basis for indeterminate egg production in female fishes. In: Creswell RL, editor. Proceedings of the Fifty-Third Annual Gulf and Caribbean Fisheries Institute. Fort Pierce: Mississippi/Alabama Sea Grant Consortium; 2002. pp. 537-552

[17] Lo Nostro F, Grier H, Andreone L, Guerrero GA. Involvement of the gonadal germinal epithelium during sex reversal and seasonal testicular cycling in the protogynous swamp eel, *Synbranchus marmoratus* Bloch 1795 (Teleostei, Synbranchidae). Journal of Morphology. 2003;**257**(1):107-126. DOI: 10.1002/jmor.10105

[18] Brown-Peterson NJ, Wyanski DM, Saborido-Rey F, Macewicz BJ, Lowerre-Barbieri SK. A standardized terminology for describing reproductive development in fishes. Marine and Coastal Fisheries. 2011;**3**(1):52-70. DOI: 10.1080/19425120.2011.555724

[19] Quagio-Grassiotto I, Grier H, Mazzoni TS, Nóbrega RH, Amorim JPA. Activity of the ovarian germinal epithelium in the freshwater catfish, *Pimelodus maculatus* (Teleostei: Ostariophysi: Siluriformes): Germline cysts, follicle formation and oocyte development. Journal of Morphology. 2011;**272**(11):1290-1306. DOI: 10.1002/jmor.10981

[20] Miranda ACL, Bazzoli N, Rizzo E, Sato Y. Ovarian follicular atresia in two teleost species: A histological and ultrastructural study. Tissue and Cell. 1999;**31**(5):480-488. DOI: 10.1054/tice.1999.0045

[21] Wallace RA, Sellman K. Cellular and dynamic aspects of oocyte growth in teleosts. Integrative and Comparative Biology. 1981;**21**(2):325-343. DOI: 10.1093/icb/21.2.325

[22] Dias JF, Peres-Rios E, Chaves PTC, Rossi-Wongtschowski CLD. Análise macroscópica dos ovários de teleósteos: problemas de classificação e recomendações de procedimentos. Revista Brasileira de Biologia. 1998;**58**(1):55-69

[23] Honji RM, Vaz-dos-Santos AM, Rossi-Wongtschowski CLDB. Identification of the stages of ovarian maturation of the argentine hake Merluccius hubbsi Marini, 1933 (Teleostei: Merlucciidae): Advantages and disadvantages of the use of the macroscopic and microscopic scales. Neotropical Ichthyology. 2006;**4**(3):329-337. DOI: 10.1590/S1679-62252006000300004

[24] Lowerre-Barbieri SK, Brown-Peterson NJ, Murua H, Tomkiewicz J, Wyanski DM, Saborido-Rey F. Emerging issues and methodological advances in fisheries reproductive biology. Marine and Coastal Fisheries: Management and Ecosystem Science. 2011;**3**(1):32-51. DOI: 10.1080/19425120.2011.555725

[25] Coward K, Bromage NR. Reproductive physiology of female tilapia broodstock. Reviews in Fish Biology and Fisheries. 2000;**10**(1):1-25. DOI: 10.1023/A:1008942318272

[26] Tyler CR, Sumpter JP. Oocyte growth and development in teleosts. Reviews in Fish Biology and Fisheries. 1996;**6**(3):287-318. DOI: 10.1007/BF00122584

[27] Coward K, Bromage NR, Hibbitt O, Parrington J. Gamete physiology,

fertilization and egg activation in teleost fish. Reviews in Fish Biology and Fisheries. 2002;**12**(1):33-58. DOI: 10.1023/A:1022613404123

[28] Grier HJ. Ovarian germinal epithelium and folliculogenesis in the common snook, *Centropomus undecimalis* (Teleostei: Centropomidae). Journal of Morphology. 2000;**243**(3):265-281. DOI: 10.1002/%28SICI%291097-4687%28200003%29243%3A3<265%3A%3AAID-JMOR4>3.0.CO%3B2-I

[29] Grier JH, Uribe-Aranzábal MC, Patiño R. The ovary, folliculogenesis and oogenesis in teleosts. In: Jamieson BJM, editor. Reproductive Biology and Phylogeny of Fishes (Agnathans and Bony Fishes) Phylogeny Reproductive System Viviparity Spermatozoa. Enfield: Science Publishers; 2009. pp. 25-84

[30] Stehr CM, Hawkes JW. The comparative ultrastructure of the egg membrane and associated pore structures in the starry flounder, *Platichthys stellatus* (Pallas), and pink salmon, *Oncorhynchus gorbuscha* (Walbaum). Cell and Tissue Research. 1979;**202**(3):347-356. DOI: 10.1007/BF00220430

[31] Francolini M, Lora Lamia C, Bonsignorio C, Cotelli F. Oocyte development and egg envelope formation in *Oreochromis niloticus*, a mouth-brooding cichlid fish. Journal of Submicroscopic Cytology and Pathology. 2003;**35**(1):49-60

[32] Hubbard JW. The yolk nucleus in *Cynematogaster aggregatus* Gibbons. Proceedings of the American Philosophical Society. 1894;**33**(144):74-83

[33] Yamamoto K. Studies on the formation of fish eggs. Annual cycle in the development of the ovarian eggs in the flounder, *Lipsetta obscura*. Journal of the Faculty of Science, Hokkaido University, Series IV—Zoology. 1956;**12**(3):362-373

[34] Agostinho AA, Suzuki HI, Sampaio AA, Borges JD. Índice de atividade reprodutiva: uma proposta para avaliação da atividade reprodutiva em peixes. In: Encontro Brasileiro De Ictiologia, Abstract. Maringá – PR; 1991. p. 53

[35] Agostinho AA, Mendes VP, Suzuki HI, Canzi C. Avaliação da atividade reprodutiva da comunidade de peixes dos primeiros quilômetros a jusante do reservatório de Itaipu. Revista UNIMAR. 1993;**15**(suppl):175-189

[36] Munro AD. General introduction. In: Munro AD, Scott AP, Lam TJ, editors. Reproductive Seasonality in Teleosts: Environmental Influences. Florida: CRC Press; 1990. pp. 1-11

[37] Munro AD. Tropical freshwater fish. In: Munro AD, Scott AP, Lam TJ, editors. Reproductive Seasonality in Teleosts: Environmental Influences. Florida: CRC Press; 1990. pp. 145-239

[38] Suzuki HI, Vazzoler AEAM, Marques EE, Lizama MAP, Inada P. Reproductive ecology of the fish assemblages. In: Thomaz SM, Agostinho AA, Hahn NS, editors. The Upper Paraná River and Its Floodplain: Physical Aspects, Ecology and Conservation. Leiden: Backhuys Publishers; 2004. pp. 271-291

[39] Nørrevanag A. Electron microscopic morphology of oogenesis. International Review of Cytology. 1968;**23**:113-186. DOI: 10.1016/S0074-7696(08)60271-5

[40] Anderson H. Comparative aspects of ultrastructure of female gamete. International Review of Cytology. 1974;**4**(Suppl):1-70

[41] Huebner E. Oocyte-follicle cell interaction during normal

oogenesis and atresia in an insect. Journal of Ultrastructure Research. 1981;**74**(1):95-104. DOI: 10.1016/S0022-5320(81)80112-8

[42] Biliński S, Klag J. GAP junctions between oocyte and follicle cells in Acerentomon sp. (Insecta, Protura). International Journal of Invertebrate Reproduction and Development. 1982;**5**(6):331-335. DOI: 10.1080/01651269.1982.10553486

[43] Khan HR, Saleuddin ASM. Cell contacts between follicle cells and oocyte of Helisoma (Mollusca, Pulmonata). Journal of Morphology. 1983;**177**(3):319-328. DOI: 10.1002/jmor.1051770308

[44] Anderson E, Albertini DF. GAP junctions between the oocyte and companion follicle cells in the mammalian ovary. The Journal of Cell Biology. 1976;**71**(2):680-686. DOI: 10.1083/jcb.71.2.680

[45] Toshimori K, Yasuzumi F. Tight junctions between ovarian follicle cells in the teleost (*Plecoglossus altivelis*). Journal of Ultrastructure Research. 1979;**67**(1):73-78. DOI: 10.1016/S0022-5320(79)80019-2

[46] Kobayashi W. Communications of oocyte-granulosa cells in the Chum salmon ovary detected by transmission electron microscopy. Development, Growth and Differentiation. 1985;**27**(5):553-561. DOI: 10.1111/j.1440-169X.1985.00553.x

[47] Larsen WJ, Wert SE. Roles of cell junctions in gametogenesis and in early embryonic development. Tissue and Cell. 1988;**20**(6):809-848. DOI: 10.1016/0040-8166(88)90025-0

[48] White TW, Paul D. Genetic diseases and gene knockouts reveal diverse connexin functions. Annual Review of Physiology. 1999;**61**:283-310. DOI: 10.1146/annurev.physiol.61.1.283

[49] Bolamba D, Patiño R, Yoshizaki G, Thomas P. Changes in homologous and heterelogous gap junction contacts during maturation-inducing hormone-dependent meiotic resumption in ovarian follicles of Atlantic croaker. General and Comparative Endocrinology. 2003;**131**(3):291-295. DOI: 10.1016/S0016-6480(03)00015-7

[50] Patiño R, Thomas P, Yoshizaki G. Ovarian follicle maturation and ovulation: An integrated perspective. Fish Physiology and Biochemistry. 2003;**28**:305-308. DOI: 10.1023/B:FISH.0000030565.74702.0a

[51] Caveney S. The role of GAP junctions in development. Annual Review of Physiology. 1985;**47**:319-335. DOI: 10.1146/annurev.ph.47.030185.001535

[52] Friend DS, Gilula NB. Variations in tight and GAP junctions in mammalian tissues. The Journal of Cell Biology. 1972;**53**(3):758-776. DOI: 10.1083/jcb.53.3.758

[53] Staehelin LA. Structure and function of intercellular junctions. International Review of Cytology. 1974;**39**:191-283. DOI: 10.1016/S0074-7696(08)60940-7

[54] Rodewald M, Herr D, Fraser HM, Hack G, Kreienberg R, Wulff C. Regulation of tight junction proteins occludin and claudin-5 in the primate ovary during the ovulatory cycle and after inhibition of vascular endothelial growth factor. Molecular Human Reproduction. 2007;**13**(11):781-789. DOI: 10.1093/molehr/gam066

[55] Dejana E. Endothelial cell–cell junctions: Happy together. Nature Reviews. Molecular Cell Biology. 2004;**5**(4):261-270. DOI: 10.1038/nrm1357

[56] Schneeberger EE, Lynch RD. The tight junction: A multifunctional complex. American Journal of Physiology. Cell Physiology.

2004;**286**(6):C1213-C1228. DOI: 10.1152/ajpcell.00558.2003

[57] Morita K, Sasaki H, Furuse M, Tsukita S. Endothelial claudin: Claudin-5/TMVCF constitutes tight junction strands in endothelial cells. The Journal of Cell Biology. 1999;**147**(1): 185-194. DOI: 10.1083/jcb.147.1.185

[58] Morita K, Sasaki H, Furuse K, Furuse M, Tsukita S, Miyachi Y. Expression of claudin-5 in dermal vascular endothelia. Experimental Dermatology. 2003;**12**(3):289-295. DOI: 10.1034/j.1600-0625.2003.120309.x

[59] Peppi M, Ghabriel MN. Tissue-specific expression of the tight junction proteins claudins and occludin in the rat salivary glands. Journal of Anatomy. 2004;**205**(4):257-266. DOI: 10.1111/j.0021-8782.2004.00332.x

[60] Cunningham BA, Edelman GE. Structure, expression, and cell surface modulation of cell adhesion molecules. In: Edelman GM, Cunningham BA, Thiery JP, editors. Morphoregulatory Molecules. New York: John Wiley and Sons; 1990. pp. 9-40

[61] Geiger B, Ayalon O. Cadherins. Annual Review of Cell Biology. 1992;**8**:307-332. DOI: 10.1146/annurev.cb.08.110192.001515

[62] Cerdà J, Reidenbach S, Prätzel S, Franke WW. Cadherin-catenin complexes during zebrafish oogenesis: Heterotypic junctions between oocytes and follicle cells. Biology of Reproduction. 1999;**61**(3):692-704. DOI: 10.1095/biolreprod61.3.692

[63] Gumbiner BM. Proteins associated with the cytoplasmic surface of adhesion molecules. Neuron. 1993;**11**(4):551-564. DOI: 10.1016/0896-6273(93)90068-3

[64] Knudsen KA, Soler AP, Johnson KR, Wheelock MJ. Interaction of α-actinin with the cadherin cell–cell adhesion complex via α-catenin. The Journal of Cell Biology. 1995;**130**(1):67-77. DOI: 10.1083/jcb.130.1.67

[65] Albelda SM, Buck CA. Integrins and other cell adhesion molecules. The FASEB Journal. 1990;**4**(11):2868-2880. DOI: 10.1096/fasebj.4.11.2199285

[66] Geiger B, Ginsberg D. The cytoplasmic domain of adherens-type junctions. Cell Motility and Cytoskeleton. 1991;**20**(1):1-6. DOI: 10.1002/cm.970200102

[67] Edelman GR. A golden age for adhesion. Cell Communication and Adhesion. 1993;**1**(1):1-7. DOI: 10.3109/15419069309095677

[68] Gall L, Picheral B, Gounon P. Cytochemical evidence for the presence of intermediate filaments and microfilaments in the egg of *Xenopus laevis*. Biology of the Cell. 1983;**47**:331-342

[69] Schroeder TE, Otto JJ. Snoods: A periodic network containing cytokeratin in the cortex of starfish oocytes. Developmental Biology. 1991;**144**(2):240-247. DOI: 10.1016/0012-1606(91)90418-3

[70] Ball EH, Singer SJ. Mitochondria are associated with microtubules and not with intermediate filaments in cultured fibroblasts. Proceedings of the National Academy of Sciences of the United States of America. 1982;**79**(1):123-126. DOI: 10.1073/pnas.79.1.123

[71] Rizzo E, Godinho HP, Sato Y. Short-term storage of oocytes from the neotropical teleost fish *Prochilodus marggravii*. Theriogenology. 2003;**60**(6):1059-1070. DOI: 10.1016/S0093-691X(03)00108-0

[72] Franke WW, Schmid E, Schiller DL, Winter S, Jarasch ED, Moll R, et al. Differentiation-related

patterns of expression of proteins of intermediate-size filaments in tissue and cultured cells. Cold Spring Harbor Symposia on Quantitative Biology. 1982;**46**:431-453. DOI: 10.1101/SQB.1982.046.01.041

[73] Lazarides E. Intermediate filaments: A chemically heterogeneous, developmentally regulated class of proteins. Annual Review of Biochemistry. 1982;**51**:219-250. DOI: 10.1146/annurev.bi.51.070182.001251

[74] Jackson BW, Grund C, Schmid E, Butki K, Franke WW, Ilimensee K. Formation of cytoskeletal elements during mouse embryogenesis: Intermediate filaments of the cytokeratin type and desmosomes in preimplantation embryos. Differentiation. 1980;**17**(1-3):161-179. DOI: 10.1111/j.1432-0436.1980.tb01093.x

[75] Osborn M, Geisler N, Shaw G, Sharp G, Weber K. Intermediate filaments. Cold Spring Harbor Symposia on Quantitative Biology. 1982;**46**:413-429. DOI: 10.1101/SQB.1982.046.01.040

[76] Godsave SF, Wylie CC, Lane EB, Anderton BH. Intermediate filaments in the Xenopus oocyte: The appearance and distribution of cytokeratin-containing filaments. Journal of Embryology and Experimental Morphology. 1984;**83**:157-167

[77] Franke WW, Rathke PC, Seib E, Trendelenburg MF, Osborn M, Weber K. Distribution and mode of arrangement of microfilamentous structures and actin in the cortex of the amphibian oocyte. Cytobiologie. 1976;**14**(1):111-130

[78] Bluemink JG. Effects of cytochalasin-b on surface contractility and cell junction formation during egg cleavage in *Xenopus laevis*. Cytobiologie. 1971;**3**:176-187

[79] Bluemink JG. Cytokinesis and cytochalasin-induced furrow regression in the first-cleavage zygote of *Xenopus laevis*. Cell and Tissue Research. 1971;**121**(1):102-126

[80] Otto JJ, Schroeder TE. Microtubule arrays in the cortex and near the germinal vesicle of immature starfish oocytes. Developmental Biology. 1984;**101**(2):274-281. DOI: 10.1016/0012-1606(84)90141-6

[81] Lessman CA, Habibi HR, Macrae TH. Effect of microtubule reactive drugs on steroid- and centrifugation-induced germinal vesicle migration during goldfish oocyte meiosis. The Biology of the Cell. 1988;**64**(3):293-299. DOI: 10.1016/0248-4900(88)90003-2

[82] Raven CHP. Oogenesis. The Storage of Developmental Information. New York: Pergamon Press; 1961. 274 p

[83] Caron JM, Berlin RD. Interaction of microtubule proteins with phospholipid vesicles. The Journal of Cell Biology. 1979;**81**(3):665-671. DOI: 10.1083/jcb.81.3.665

[84] Guraya SS. Recent advances in the morphology, cytochemistry and function of Balbiani's vitelline body in animal oocytes. International Review of Cytology. 1979;**59**:249-321. DOI: 10.1016/S0074-7696(08)61664-2

[85] Klausner RD, Kumar N, Weinstein JN, Blumenthal R, Flavin M. Interaction of tubulin with membrane vesicles. I. Association with vesicles at the phase transition. The Journal of Biological Chemistry. 1981;**256**(11):5879-5885

[86] Tourte M, Mignotte F, Mounolou J. Heterogenous distribution and replication activity of mitochondria in *Xenopus laevis* oocytes. European Journal of Cell Biology. 1984;**34**(1):171-178

[87] Paleček J, Habrová V, Nedvídek J, Romanovský A. Dynamics of tubulin structures in *Xenopus laevis* oogenesis. Journal of Embryology and Experimental Morphology. 1985;**87**:75-86

[88] Khodjakov A, Rieder CL. The sudden recruitment of g-tubulin to the centrosome at the onset of mitosis and its dynamic exchange throughout the cell cycle, do not require microtubules. The Journal of Cell Biology. 1999;**146**(3):585-596. DOI: 10.1083/jcb.146.3.585

[89] Santella L, Puppo A, Chun JT. The role of the actin cytoskeleton in calcium signaling in starfish oocytes. The International Journal of Developmental Biology. 2008;**52**(5-6):571-584. DOI: 10.1387/ijdb.072560ls

[90] Welch MD, Mallavarpu A, Rosenblatt J, Mitchison TJ. Actin dynamics in vivo. Current Opinion in Cell Biology. 1997;**99**(1):54-61. DOI: 10.1016/S0955-0674(97)80152-4

[91] Barnett DK, Clayton MK, Kimura J, Bavister BD. Glucose and phosphate toxicity in hamster preimplantation embryos involves distribution of cellular organization, including distribution of active mitochondria. Molecular Reproduction and Development. 1997;**48**(2):227-237. DOI: 10.1002/%28SICI%291098-2795%28199710%2948%3A2<227%3A%3AAID-MRD10>3.0.CO%3B2-V

[92] Valderrama F, Babià T, Ayala I, Kok JW, Renau-Pigueras J, Egea G. Actin microfilaments are essential for the cytological position and morphology of the golgi complex. European Journal of Cell Biology. 1998;**76**(1):9-17. DOI: 10.1016/S0171-9335(98)80012-5

[93] Terasaki M. Redistribution of cytoplasmic components during germinal vesicle breakdown in starfish oocytes. Journal of Cell Science. 1994;**107**(Pt7):1797-1805

[94] Berg L, Wessel G. Cortical granules of the sea urchin translocate early in oocyte maturation. Development. 1997;**124**(9):1845-1850

[95] Cantiello HF. Role of actin filament organization in cell volume and ion channel regulation. The Journal of Experimental Zoology. 1997;**279**(5):425-435. DOI: 10.1002/%28SICI%291097-010X%2819971201%29279%3A5<425%3A%3AAID-JEZ4>3.0.CO%3B2-Q

[96] Wang WH, Abeydeera LR, Prather RS, Day BN. Polymerization of nonfilamentous actin into microfilaments is an important process for porcine oocyte maturation and early embryo development. Biology of Reproduction. 2000;**62**(5):1177-1183. DOI: 10.1095/biolreprod62.5.1177

[97] Lange K, Brandt U. Calcium storage and release properties of F-actin: Evidence for the involvement of F-actin in cellular calcium signaling. FEBS Letters. 1996;**395**(2-3):137-142. DOI: 10.1016/0014-5793(96)01025-3

[98] Janmey PA. The cytoskeleton and cell signaling: Component localization and mechanical coupling. Physiological Reviews. 1998;**78**(3):763-781. DOI: 10.1152/physrev.1998.78.3.763

[99] Schroeder TE, Stricker SA. Morphological changes during maturation of starfish oocytes: Surface ultrastructure and cortical actin. Developmental Biology. 1983;**98**(2):373-384. DOI: 10.1016/0012-1606(83)90366-4

[100] Otto JJ, Schroeder TE. Assembly-disassembly of actin bundles in starfish oocytes: An analysis of actin-associated proteins in the isolated cortex. Developmental Biology. 1984;**101**(2):263-273. DOI: 10.1016/0012-1606(84)90140-4

[101] Santella L, De Riso L, Gragnaniello G, Kyozuka K. Cortical granule translocation during maturation of starfish oocytes requires cytoskeletal rearrangement triggered by InsP3-mediated Ca2+ release. Experimental Cell Research. 1999;**248**(2):567-574. DOI: 10.1006/excr.1999.4425

[102] Morais RDVS, Thomé RG, Lemos FS, Bazzoli N, Rizzo E. Autophagy and apoptosis interplay during follicular atresia in fish ovary: A morphological and immunocytochemical study. Cell and Tissue Research. 2012;**347**(2):467-478. DOI: 10.1007/s00441-012-1327-6

[103] Korsnes MS, Hetland DL, Espenes A, Aune T. Cleavage of tensin during cytoskeleton disruption in YTX-induced apoptosis. Toxicology In Vitro. 2007;**21**(1):9-15. DOI: 10.1016/j.tiv.2006.07.012

[104] Byskov AG. Follicular atresia. In: Jones RE, editor. The Vertebrate Ovary. New York: Plenum Press; 1978. pp. 533-562

[105] Saidapur SK. Follicular atresia in the ovaries of non mammalian vertebrates. International Review of Cytology. 1978;**54**:225-244. DOI: 10.1016/S0074-7696(08)60169-2

[106] Nagahama Y. The functional morphology of the teleost gonad. In: Hoar WS, Randall DJ, Donaldson EM, editors. Fish Physiology, Vol. IX, Chapter 6. Reproduction, Part A: Endocrine Tissues and Hormones. Cambridge: Academic Press; 1983. pp. 223-275. DOI: 10.1016/s1546-5098(08)60290-3

[107] Nagahama Y. Endocrine regulation of gametogenesis in fish. The International Journal of Developmental Biology. 1994;**38**(2):217-229

[108] Mylonas CC, Woods LC III, Zohar Y. Cyto-histological examination of post-vitellogenesis and final oocyte maturation in captive-reared striped bass. Journal of Fish Biology. 1997;**50**(1):34-49. DOI: 10.1111/j.1095-8649.1997.tb01338.x

[109] Guimarães CA, Linden R. Programmed cell deaths. Apoptosis and alternative deathstyles. European Journal of Biochemistry. 2004;**271**(9):1638-1650. DOI: 10.1111/j.1432-1033.2004.04084.x

[110] Hoar WS. Reproduction. In: Hoar W, Randall DJ, editors. Fish Physiology. London: Academic Press; 1969. pp. 1-72

[111] Ganeco LN, Nakaghi LSO, Urbinati EC, Dumont Neto R, Vasques LH. Análise morfológica do desenvolvimento ovocitário de piracanjuba, Brycon orbignyanus, durante o ciclo reprodutivo. Boletim do Instituto de Pesca—São Paulo. 2001;**27**(2):131-138

[112] Janz DM, Van der Kraak G. Suppression of apoptosis by gonadotropin 17beta-estradiol and epidermal growth factor in rainbow trout preovulatory ovarian follicles. General and Comparative Endocrinology. 1997;**105**(2):186-193. DOI: 10.1006/gcen.1996.6820

[113] Wood AW, Van der Kraak GJ. Apoptosis and ovarian function: Novel perspectives from the teleosts. Biology of Reproduction. 2001;**64**(1):264-271. DOI: 10.1095/biolreprod64.1.264

[114] Drummond CD, Bazzoli N, Rizzo E, Sato Y. Postovulatory follicle: A model for experimental studies of programmed cell death or apoptosis in teleost. The Journal of Experimental Zoology. 2000;**287**(2):176-182. DOI: 10.1002/1097-010X%2820000701%29287%3A2<176%3A%3AAID-JEZ8>3.0.CO%3B2-2

[115] Thomé RG, Santos HB, Arantes FP, Prado PS, Domingos FFT, Sato Y, et al. Regression of post-ovulatory follicles in

Prochilodus costatus Valenciennes, 1850 (Characiformes, Prochilodontidae). Brazilian Journal of Morphological Sciences. 2006;**23**(3-4):495-500

[116] Santos HB, Thomé RG, Arantes FP, Sato Y, Bazzoli N, Rizzo E. Ovarian follicular atresia is mediated by heterophagy, autophagy, and apoptosis in *Prochilodus argenteus* and *Leporinus taeniatus* (Teleostei: Characiformes). Theriogenology. 2008;**70**(9):1449-1460. DOI: 10.1016/j.theriogenology.2008.06.091

[117] Agulleiro MJ, André M, Morais S, Cerdà J, Babin PJ. High transcript level of fatty acid-binding protein 11 but not of very low-density lipoprotein receptor is correlated to ovarian follicle atresia in a teleost fish (*Solea senegalensis*). Biology of Reproduction. 2007;**77**(3):504-516. DOI: 10.1095/biolreprod.107.061598

[118] Rajalakshmi M. Atresia of oocytes and ruptured follicles in *Gobius giuris* (Hamilton-Buchanan). General and Comparative Endocrinology. 1966;**6**(3):378-385. DOI: 10.1016/S0016-6480(66)80025-4

[119] Rizzo E, Bazzoli N. Follicular atresia in curimatá-pioa *Prochilodus affinis* Reinhardt, 1874 (Pisces, Characiformes). Revista Brasileira de Biologia. 1995;**55**:697-703

[120] Linares-Casenave J, Van Eenennaam JP, Doroshov SI. Ultrastructural and histological observations on temperature-induced follicular ovarian atresia in the white sturgeon. Journal of Applied Ichthyology. 2002;**18**:382-390. DOI: 10.1046/j.1439-0426.2002.00369.x

[121] Santos HB, Rizzo E, Bazzoli N, Sato Y, Moro L. Ovarian regression and apoptosis in the South American teleost *Leporinus taeniatus* Lütken (Characiformes, Anostomidae) from the São Francisco Basin. Journal of Fish Biology. 2005;**67**(5):1446-1459. DOI: 10.1111/j.1095-8649.2005.00854.x

[122] Quintana CF, Cohene TB, Arbués R, Domitrovic H, González J. Follicular atresia in ovaries of *Prochilodus lineatus*. International Journal of Morphology. 2012;**30**:1301-1308. DOI: 10.4067/S0717-95022012000400008

[123] Senerat S, Kettratad J, Jiraungkoorskul W. Classification stages of novel atretic structure in short mackerel Rastrelliger brachysoma (Bleeker, 1851) from the Upper Gulf of Thailand. Songklanakarin Journal of Science and Technology. 2015;**37**:569-573

[124] Cassel M, Camargo MP, Jesus LWO, Borella MI. Involution processes of follicular atresia and post-ovulatory complex in a characid fish ovary: A study of apoptosis and autophagy pathways. Journal of Molecular Histology. 2017;**48**(3):243-257. DOI: 10.1007/s10735-017-9723-6

[125] Janz DM, McMaster ME, Munkittrick KR, Van der Kraak G. Elevated ovarian follicular apoptosis and heat shock protein-70 expression in white sucker exposed to bleached kraft pulp mill effluent. Toxicology and Applied Pharmacology. 1997;**147**(2):391-398. DOI: 10.1006/taap.1997.8283

[126] Hacker G. The morphology of apoptosis. Cell and Tissue Research. 2000;**301**:5-17. DOI: 10.1007/s004410000193

[127] Huettenbrenner S, Maier S, Leisser C, Polgar D, Strasser S, Grusch M, et al. The evolution of cell death programs as prerequisites of multicellularity. Mutation Research. 2003;**543**:235-249. DOI: 10.1016/S1383-5742(02)00110-2

[128] Krumschnabel G, Podrabsky JE. Fish as model systems for the study

of vertebrate apoptosis. Apoptosis. 2009;**14**:1-21. DOI: 10.1007/s10495-008-0281-y

[129] Boone DL, Tsang BK. Caspase-3 in the rat ovary: Localization and possible role in follicular atresia and luteal regression. Biology of Reproduction. 1998;**58**:1533-1539. DOI: 10.1095/biolreprod58.6.1533

[130] Thomé RG, Santos HB, Arantes FP, Domingos FFT, Bazzoli N, Rizzo E. Dual roles for autophagy during follicular atresia in fish ovary. Autophagy. 2009;**5**(1):117-119. DOI: 10.4161/auto.5.1.7302

[131] Maiuri MC, Zalckvar E, Kimchi A, Kroemer G. Self-eating and self-killing: Crosstalk between autophagy and apoptosis. Nature Reviews. Molecular Cell Biology. 2007;**8**(9):741-752. DOI: 10.1038/nrm2239

[132] Mizushima N, Levine B, Cuervo AM, Klionsky DJ. Autophagy fights disease through cellular self-digestion. Nature. 2008;**451**(7182):1069-1075. DOI: 10.1038/nature06639

[133] Maiuri MC, Criollo A, Kroemer G. Crosstalk between apoptosis and autophagy within the Beclin 1 interactome. The EMBO Journal. 2010;**29**(3):515-516. DOI: 10.1038/emboj.2009.377

[134] Thomé R, Santos HB, Sato Y, Rizzo E, Bazzoli N. Distribution of laminin beta2, collagen type IV, fibronectin and MMP-9 in ovaries of the teleost fish. Journal of Molecular Histology. 2010;**41**(4-5):215-224. DOI: 10.1007/s10735-010-9281-7

[135] Drevinick PE, Sandheinrich MB, Oris JT. Increased ovarian follicular apoptosis in fathead minnows (*Pimephales promelas*) exposed to dietary methylmercury. Aquatic Toxicology. 2006;**79**(1):49-54. DOI: 10.1016/j.aquatox.2006.05.007

[136] Saito D, Morinaga C, Aoki Y, Nakamura S, Mitani H, Furutani-Seiki M, et al. Proliferation of germ cells during gonadal sex differentiation in medaka: Insights from germ cell-depleted mutant zenzai. Developmental Biology. 2007;**310**(2):280-290. DOI: 10.1016/j.ydbio.2007.07.039

[137] Krysko DV, Diez-Fraile A, Criel G, Svistunov AA, Vandenabeele P, D'Herde K. Life and death of female gametes during oogenesis and folliculogenesis. Apoptosis. 2008;**13**(9):1065-1087. DOI: 10.1007/s10495-008-0238-1

[138] Tokarz RR. Oogonial proliferation, oogenesis and folliculogenesis in nonmammalian vertebrates. In: Jones RE, editor. The Vertebrate Ovary. Comparative Biology and Evolution. New York: Plenum Press; 1978. pp. 145-179

[139] Jalabert B. Particularities of reproduction and oogenesis in teleost fish compared to mammals. Reproduction Nutrition Development. 2005;**45**(3):261-279. DOI: 10.1051/rnd:2005019

[140] Nakamura S, Kobayashi K, Nishimura T, Tanaka M. Ovarian germline stem cells in the teleost fish, medaka (*Oryzias latipes*). International Journal of Biological Sciences. 2011;**7**(4):403-409. DOI: 10.7150/ijbs.7.403

[141] Sriramulu V, Rajalakshmi M. Origin of a new crop of oocytes in *Gobius giuris* (Hamilton-Buchanan). Zeitschrift für Mikroskopisch-Anatomische Forschung. 1966;**75**(1):64-73

[142] Billard R. The reproductive cycle of male and female brown trout (Salmo trutta fario): A quantitative study. Reproduction Nutrition Development. 1987;**27**(1A):29-44. DOI: 10.1051/rnd:19870104

[143] Selman K, Wallace RA, Sarka QIX. Stages of oocyte development in the zebrafish, *Brachydanio rerio*. Journal of

Morphology. 1993;**218**(2):203-224. DOI: 10.1002/jmor.1052180209

[144] Curry TE, Osteen KG. The matrix metalloproteinase system: Changes, regulation, and impact throughout the ovarian and uterine reproductive cycle. Endocrine Reviews. 2003;**24**(4): 428-465. DOI: 10.1210/er.2002-0005

[145] Larreta-Garde V, Berry H. Modeling extracellular matrix degradation balance with proteinase/ transglutaminase cycle. Journal of Theoretical Biology. 2002;**217**(1): 105-124. DOI: 10.1006/jtbi.2002.3010

[146] Price JT, Bonovich MT, Kohn EC. The biochemistry of cancer dissemination. Critical Reviews in Biochemistry and Molecular Biology. 1997;**32**(3):175-253. DOI: 10.3109/10409239709082573

[147] Basbaum CB, Werb Z. Focalized proteolysis: Spatial and temporal regulation of extracellular matrix degradation at the cell surface. Current Opinion in Cell Biology. 1996;**8**(5):731-738. DOI: 10.1016/ S0955-0674(96)80116-5

[148] Schalburg KR, Cooper GA, Yazawa R, Davidson WS, Koop BF. Microarray analysis reveals differences in expression of cell surface and extracellular matrix components during development of the trout ovary and testis. Comparative Biochemistry and Physiology. 2008;**3**(1):78-90. DOI: 10.1016/j.cbd.2007.10.001

[149] Dustin ML, De Fougerolles AR. Reprogramming T cells: The role of extracellular matrix in coordination of T cell activation and migration. Current Opinion in Immunology. 2001;**13**(3):286-290. DOI: 10.1016/ S0952-7915(00)00217-X

[150] Witte MB, Barbul A. General principles of wound healing. The Surgical Clinics of North America. 1997;**77**(3):509-528. DOI: 10.1016/ S0039-6109(05)70566-1

[151] Davis GE, Bayless KJ, Davis MJ, Meininger GA. Regulation of tissue injury responses by the exposure of matricryptic sites within extracellular matrix molecules. The American Journal of Pathology. 2000;**156**(5):1489-1498. DOI: 10.1016/S0002-9440(10)65020-1

[152] Hay ED. Collagen and embryonic development. In: Hay ED, editor. Cell Biology of Extracellular Matrix. New York: PlenumPress; 1981. pp. 379-409

[153] Perris R, Perissinotto D. Role of the extracellular matrix during neural crest cell migration. Mechanisms of Development. 2000;**95**(1-2):3-21. DOI: 10.1016/S0925-4773(00)00365-8

[154] Hulboy DL, Rudolph LA, Matrisian LM. Matrix metalloproteinases as mediators of reproductive function. Molecular Human Reproduction. 1997;**3**(1):27-45

[155] Irving-Rodgers HF, Rodgers RJ. Extracellular matrix in ovarian follicular development and disease. Cell and Tissue Research. 2005;**322**(1):89-98. DOI: 10.1007/s00441-005-0042-y

[156] Oksjoki S, Sallinen S, Vuorio E, Anttila L. Cyclic expression of mRNA transcripts for connective tissue components in the mouse ovary. Molecular Human Reproduction. 1999;**5**(9):803-808. DOI: 10.1093/ molehr/5.9.803

[157] Rodgers RJ, Lavranos TC, Van Wezel IL, Irving-Rodgers HF. Development of the ovarian follicular epithelium. Molecular and Cellular Endocrinology. 1999;**151**(1-2):171-179. DOI: 10.1016/S0303-7207(99)00087-8

[158] Skinner MK, Tung PS, Fritz IB. Cooperativity between Sertoli cells and testicular peritubular cells in

the production and deposition of extracellular matrix components. The Journal of Cell Biology. 1985;**100**(6):1941-1947. DOI: 10.1083/jcb.100.6.1941

[159] Rodgers RJ, Irving-Rodgers HF, Russell DL. Extracellular matrix of the developing ovarian follicle. Reproduction. 2003;**126**(4):415-424

[160] Sternilicht MD, Werb Z. How matrix metalloproteinase regulate cell behavior. Annual Review of Cell and Developmental Biology. 2001;**17**(1):463-516. DOI: 10.1146/annurev.cellbio.17.1.463

[161] Smith MF, Ricke WA, Bakke LJ, Dow MPD, Smith GW. Ovarian tissue remodeling: Role of matrix metalloproteinases and their inhibitors. Molecular and Cellular Endocrinology. 2002;**191**(1):45-56. DOI: 10.1016/S0303-7207(02)00054-0

[162] Ogiwara K, Takano N, Shinohara M, Murakami M, Takahashi T. Gelatinase A and membrane-type matrix metalloproteinases 1 and 2 are responsible for follicle rupture during ovulation in the medaka. Proceedings of the National Academy of Sciences of the United States of America. 2005;**102**(24):8442-8447. DOI: 10.1073/pnas.0502423102

[163] Berkholtz CB, Lai BE, Woodruff TK, Shea LD. Distribution of extracellular matrix proteins type I collagen, type IV collagen, fibronectin, and laminin in mouse folliculogenesis. Histochemistry and Cell Biology. 2006;**126**(5):583-592. DOI: 10.1007/s00418-006-0194-1

[164] Carnegie JA. Secretion of fibronectin by rat granulosa cells occurs primarily during early follicular development. Journal of Reproduction and Fertility. 1990;**89**(2):579-589. DOI: 10.1530/jrf.0.0890579

[165] Zhao Y, Luck MR. Gene expression and protein distribution of collagen, fibronectin and laminin in bovine follicles and corpora lutea. Journal of Reproduction and Fertility. 1995;**104**(1):115-123. DOI: 10.1530/jrf.0.1040115

[166] Iwahashi M, Muragaki Y, Ooshima A, Nakano R. Type VI collagen expression during growth of human ovarian follicles. Fertility and Sterility. 2000;**74**(2):343-347. DOI: 10.1016/S0015-0282(00)00618-X

Chapter 7

Reproductive Cycle of *Hexaplex princeps* (Broderip, 1833)

Verónica Mitsui Saito-Quezada, Esther Uría-Galicia, José Luis Gómez-Márquez, Ana Bertha Villaseñor-Martínez, Ma. De Lourdes Jiménez-Badillo and Isaías Hazarmabeth Salgado-Ugarte

Abstract

During two annual periods, the reproductive cycle of the gastropod *Hexaplex princeps* from Puerto Ángel, Oaxaca, Mexico was studied through gonadal histology. Sex proportion for the collected individuals was not statistically different from parity although most of the time, the number of males was slightly larger than that of females, which only outnumbered males during the spawning season. The maturity stages established for females were: (1) initial oogenesis, (2) previtellogenic maturity, (3) vitellogenic maturity, (4) maturity, (5) spawning, and (6) resting; and for males: (1) initial spermatogenesis, (2) maturity, (3) spawning, (4) onset of the rest, and (5) resting. Monthly variations of maturation stages showed that H. princeps has an annual reproductive cycle with a long period of gonadal activity. The spawning season comprised from November (females) and December (males) to March, with activity peaks in January. From March to October (females) and from May to June (males), reproduction resting occurred. Spawning was related to high chlorophyll concentrations due to the upwelling processes resulting from the winds and to the cooler sea surface temperatures occurring from November to March. This study provides baseline information that may serve to establish measures for sustainable exploitation strategies and for future aquaculture implementation of this species.

Keywords: *Hexaplex princeps*, reproductive cycle, sexual proportion, histological analysis, maturity scales

1. Introduction

Marine mollusks constitute one of the more important world fisheries representing around 10% of the total value and quantity [1]. These invertebrates have been exploited since ancient times. Recently, it has been reported that omega fatty acids, including docosahexaenoic acid (DHA) are key to brain health and most likely helped to drive the evolution of the modern human brain, when hominin ancestors consumed rich DHA marine shellfish [2]. In the world, approximately 720 gastropod species are exploited [3, 4]. In Mexico, the gastropod catch in 2013 has the 19th place with 6011 ton [5].

The gastropod *Hexaplex princeps* has a spiny shell, height from 7.6 to 15.2 cm and whirl count 6 or 9; edge of lip armed with long, hollow, and frond-like spines;

is gonochoristic and the gonad with the digestive gland occupies the visceral coils [6]; distributes from the Gulf of California to Peru inhabiting moderately shallow waters [7, 8]. The presence of this species has been reported in Panama [9]. *Hexaplex princeps* (Broderip, 1833) is captured by several artisanal fisheries of Mexico: because of its size and taste, *H. princeps* is observed with less frequency in the subtidal zone at the Tenacatita (Jalisco) coral reef in search of other prey gastropods, although can be found in rocky substrates with heavy wave action [10]. At Acapulco (Guerrero), *H. princeps* is the second major exploited species after the oyster *Striostrea prismatica* [11]. Our observations along the study period suggest that at Puerto Ángel, Oaxaca, this species is an important fishery resource as it supports around 80% of the gastropod catch for local population and tourism consumption.

In the world, artisanal fisheries are in continuous expansion due to the growing demand and increasing value of appreciated species, and thus, the fisheries effort is augmenting [12]. Under this scenario, it is advisable (if not indispensable) to gather baseline biological information that may be used to propose management measures promoting long-term sustainable resource exploitation [4].

The study of the reproductive processes in marine organisms is a fundamental biological aspect, which permits to understand their population dynamics [13]. The reproductive season is a crucial life history trait and the proper timing of breeding may be important to provide the offspring with favorable environmental conditions and to influence parental fitness [14, 15]. The analysis of the reproductive cycle of organisms permits to know the adequate moment and intensity of the capture to avoid the population depletion.

The reproduction of Muricidae members (at which *H. princeps* belongs) has been studied in several instances: the gonad cycle of *Bolinus brandaris* at the South of Portugal [16] and at the South of Tunisia [4]; in the Gulf of California, Mexico, observations on the "Black Murex" *Hexaplex nigritus* [17] and *Hexaplex erythrostomus* [18] similar oviposition. In spite of the importance of *H. princeps* as a fishery resource, there is no information on its reproductive cycle. This knowledge gap makes necessary to carry out studies on the biological cycle of this species in order to take adequate management decisions leading toward its sustainable exploitation and even its aquaculture in the future.

Thus, this study is aimed to investigate the reproductive cycle of *Hexaplex princeps*, considering sexual proportion, gonad maturation, spawning periods, and maturity stages variation in relation with the surface temperature and chlorophyll concentration along two annual periods at Puerto Angel, Oaxaca, Mexico.

2. Materials and methods

The organisms were obtained from the artisanal fishery with (as possible) monthly periodicity during two annual periods from January 2014 to November 2015. The organisms were caught with the help of two local free divers and the captain of an 8 m length vessel with a 40 HP outboard motor at depths from 5 to 15 m in rocky coast localities at the vicinity of Puerto Ángel, Oaxaca, Mexico, between 9:00 and 12:00 h local time (**Table 1**, **Figure 1**). The collecting sites were determined each date according to the atmospheric and sea conditions as well as the diver's knowledge on the species availability in the zone. Our aim was to have a representative number of specimens from the region to gather the histological information from reproductive organs and tissues.

From the caught organisms, 10–15 individuals in the interval from 8 to 12 cm in length (interval that contained more than 90% of the lengths, we collected since

Site	Latitude (N)	Longitude (W)
Punta Cometa (PC)	15° 39′ 35.4″	96° 33′ 16.5″
San Agustinillo (SA)	15° 39′ 48.6″	96° 33′ 01.0″
Playa Panteón (PP)	15° 39′ 56.1″	96° 29′ 27.1″
Aragón (Ar)	15° 39′ 38.2″	96° 31′ 46.8″
Estacahuite (Es)	15° 40′ 04.7″	96° 28′ 54.5″
Bajos de Aceite (BA)	15° 40′ 10.6″	96° 28′ 29.6″
La Mina (LM)	15° 40′ 26.7″	96° 28′ 35.7″
La Boquilla (LB)	15° 40′ 48.3″	96° 27′ 58.4″
Secretario (Sr)	15° 41′ 02.3″	96° 27′ 00.5″
Tijera (Tj)	15° 41′ 20.2″	96° 26′ 26.3″
Dominguillo (Dm)	15° 41′ 35.0″	96° 26′ 02.2″
Playita, Tembo (PT)	15° 41′ 36.1″	96° 25′ 54.3″
Temperature (SST) and chlorophyll (CL)	15° 38′ 44.9″	96° 28′ 45.0″

Table 1.
Specimen collection and environmental variables (surface sea temperature and chlorophyll) measure site geopositions.

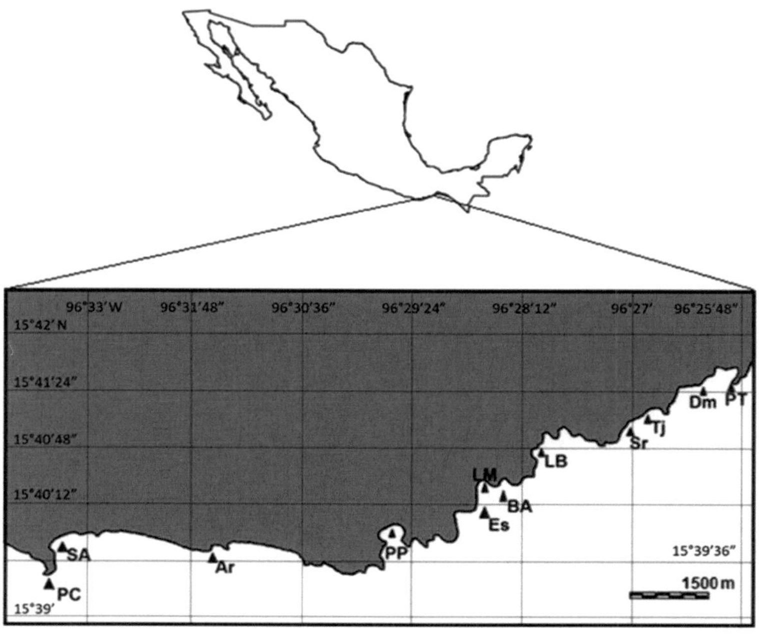

Figure 1.
Geographical location of the study area, Puerto Ángel, Oaxaca, Mexico. The collection sites are indicated: PC: Punta Cometa, SA: San Agustinillo, Ar: Aragón, PP: Playa Panteón, ES: Estacahuite. LM: La Mina, BA: Bajos de Aceite, LB: La Boquilla, Sr: Secretario, Tj: Tijera, Dm: Dominguillo, PT: Playita Tembo.

2012) were separated and their shell broken to extract the soft parts, which were fixed in formalin 10% prepared with seawater [19]. Once fixed, the specimens were transported to the Biometry and Fisheries Biology Laboratory of the Facultad de Estudios Superiores Zaragoza, UNAM, where after 48 h were washed with tap water and preserved in 70% ethylic alcohol. As there are no external characters to distinguish sex, the specimens were dissected to examine and search for the presence or absence of penis.

The sexual proportion was analyzed by means of the chi-squared goodness of fit test following the corrected Yates expression [20, 21].

The histological sections were carried out at the Histology Laboratory from the Morphology Department at the Escuela Nacional de Ciencias Biológicas, Instituto Politécnico Nacional. The alcohol-preserved specimens were dehydrated following the usual alcohol series (70–100%) and cleared in xylol before being included in paraplax and paraffin. The embedded tissues were sliced into sections of 5 μm thickness using a microtome and mounted over glass slides. The preparations were stained with the Hematoxylin-Eosin method [22] to facilitate the determination of the gonad development stages. The sections were fixed with Entalan and covered with glass slips. Finally, the preparations were observed and photographed by means of an optical microscope with attached camera.

The sea surface temperature (SST) and chlorophyll *a* of Puerto Ángel data were consulted from the GES DISC-NASA database [23, 24]. The monthly values were taken from a site in the vicinities of the Puerto Angel Bay (**Table 1**). To assess the statistical significance of the relationships between the maturity stages and the mean values of temperature and chlorophyll, two procedures were employed. In the first place, in order to clarify the pattern showed by the gonad stage percentages, a nonlinear resistant smoothing procedure was applied. The preferred smoother was the 4253eh,twice, which combines the smooth result of even span running median smoothers (4,2), the resistance of odd running medians (5,3) with end point adjustment (e), the "Hanning" weighted mean smoother (h) and the "re-roughing" (twice) step [25, 26, 27, 28, 29–32, 33].

The comparisons of the resulting time series data were performed by means of the cross-correlation analysis [34, 35, 33] between the percentages of maturity stages against the temperature and chlorophyll values. Additional cross-correlation analyses among maturity stages were made.

3. Results

3.1 Reproductive cycle

In total, 232 males and 214 females were captured. The sexual proportions throughout the study are included in **Table 2**. From the 446 individuals, 250 were analyzed for recognition and characterization of the gonad stages considering the degree of development besides the occurrence and abundance of gametes. The different gonad development stages were classified as follows: for females, six stages were established (**Table 3**, **Figure 2**). Stage 1 (S1) initial oogenesis, stage 2 (S2) previtellogenic maturity, stage 3 (S3) vitellogenic maturity, stage 4 (S4) maturity, stage 5 (S5) spawning, and finally, stage 6 (S6) resting. For males, five stages were recognized (**Table 4**, **Figure 3**). Stage 1 (S1) initial spermatogenesis, stage 2 (S2) maturity, stage 3 (S3) expulsion, stage 4 (S4) onset of rest, and stage 5 (S5) resting.

Spawning (S5) females of *H. princeps* (**Figure 4**) presented large percentages during January (60%), March (67%), and November (67%) of 2014. On the other hand, it is noted that 100% of the resting stage (S6) was registered in July. The months with larger spawning (S5) percentages during 2015 were January (60%), March (80%), and November (75%) and the months with resting (S6) larger frequency values were April (75%) and July (75%).

Collecting data and site (main)	Total	Sexo		Male:female proportion	χ^2 (Yates)	*P*
		Males	Females			
24/Jan/14 (Es)	93	40	53	1.00:1.33	1.55	0.21
21/Feb/14 (Dm)	02	02	0	—:—	0.50	0.48
21/Mar/14 (Ar)	26	16	10	1.60:1.00	0.96	0.33
25/Apr/14 (PP)	60	33	27	1.22:1.00	0.42	0.52
23/May/14 (ML)	53	27	26	1.04:1.00	0.00	1.00
15/Aug/14 (PC)	42	25	17	1.47:1.00	1.17	0.28
24/Oct/14 (PC)	13	04	09	1.00:2.25	1.23	0.27
28/Nov/14 (PT)	57	32	25	1.28:1.00	0.63	0.43
21/Dec/14 (Es)	12	07	05	1.40:1.00	0.08	0.77
30/Jan/15 (PT)	08	03	05	1.00:1.67	0.13	0.72
27/Mar/15 (PP)	07	02	05	1.00:2.50	0.57	0.45
30/Apr/15 (PP)	08	05	03	1.67:1.00	0.13	0.72
15/May/15 (LM)	08	04	04	1.00:1.00	0.13	0.72
12/Jun/15 (SA)	11	06	05	1.20:1.00	0.00	1.00
15/Jul/15 (BA)	09	06	03	2.00:1.00	0.44	0.50
21/Aug/15 (PP)	09	05	04	1.25:1.00	0.00	1.00
25/Sep/15 (PP)	10	05	05	1.00:1.00	0.10	0.75
16/Oct/15 (PP)	08	04	04	1.00:1.00	0.13	0.72
27/Nov/15 (PP)	10	06	04	1.50:1.00	0.10	0.75
Total	446	232	214	1.08:1.00	0.65	0.42

Site abbreviations according to **Table 1**.

Table 2.
Number of individuals by collecting date and site (main); sexual proportion and its statistical significance are included (χ^2 with yates correction).

Stage 1 initial oogenesis (S1)	Occurrence of developing ovogonia and oocytes, thick follicle walls
Stage 2 previtellogenic maturity (S2)	Oocytes full of yolk granules; in some oocytes, the nucleus and nucleolus are observed; follicles completely mature full of oocytes
Stage 3 vitellogenic maturity (S3)	Follicles with thin walls and developing oocytes; yolk granules are observed and yolk platelets appear
Stage 4 maturity (S4)	Follicles full of yolk granules and platelets; thin follicle walls
Stage 5 spawning (S5)	Light in the follicles is observed; follicles partially empty; follicle walls thin with some remnant oocytes
Stage 6 resting (S6)	Some resting follicles besides cells or phagocytes in thick follicle walls; conspicuous conjunctive tissue

Table 3.
Characterization of gonad development stages for females of Hexaplex princeps.

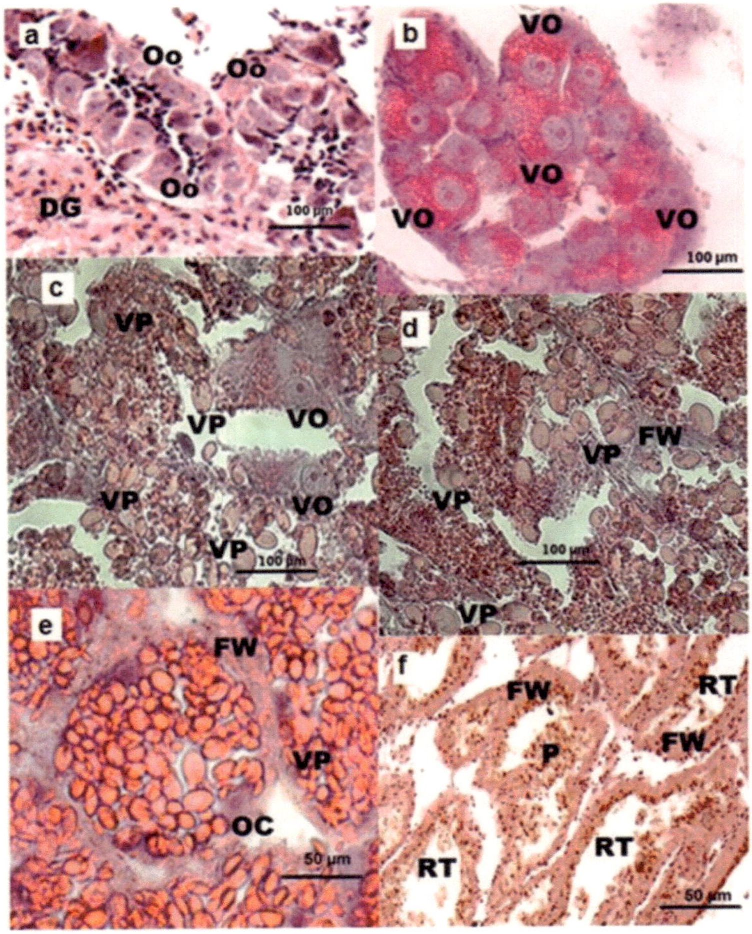

Figure 2.
Histological sections of Hexaplex princeps females showing ovary stages. a: initial oogenesis (20X), b: previtellogenic mature (10X), c: vitellogenic mature (20X), d: mature (10X), e: spawning (10X), f: resting (10X). Oo: oogonia, Oc: oocytes, DG: digestive gland, CT: connective tissue, PV: vitelline platelets, PvO: previtellogenic oocytes, VO: vitellogenic oocytes, FW: follicular wall, RO: residual oocytes, P: phagocytes.

Males of *H. princeps* (**Figure 5**) presented spawning (S3) stage in January (100%) and March (50%); the reproductive resting stage (S5) occurred in

Stage 1 initial spermatogenesis (S1)	Follicles active, developed with immature cells; small separated follicles with numerous immature cells (spermatogonia and spermatocytes), thick follicle walls
Stage 2 maturity (S2)	Follicles utterly full with a greater quantity of spermatozoids, spermatogonia, spermatocytes, and spermatids
Stage 3 spawning (S3)	Mature spermatozoids in expulsion, ciliated cylindric epithelium with foldings
Stage 4 onset of rest (S4)	Some follicles in expulsion; empty and resting follicles are observed
Stage 5 resting (S5)	Empty follicle lumen; resting follicles due to the expulsion of spermatozoids are observed; conspicuous conjunctive tissue

Table 4.
Characterization of gonad development stage for males of Hexaplex princeps.

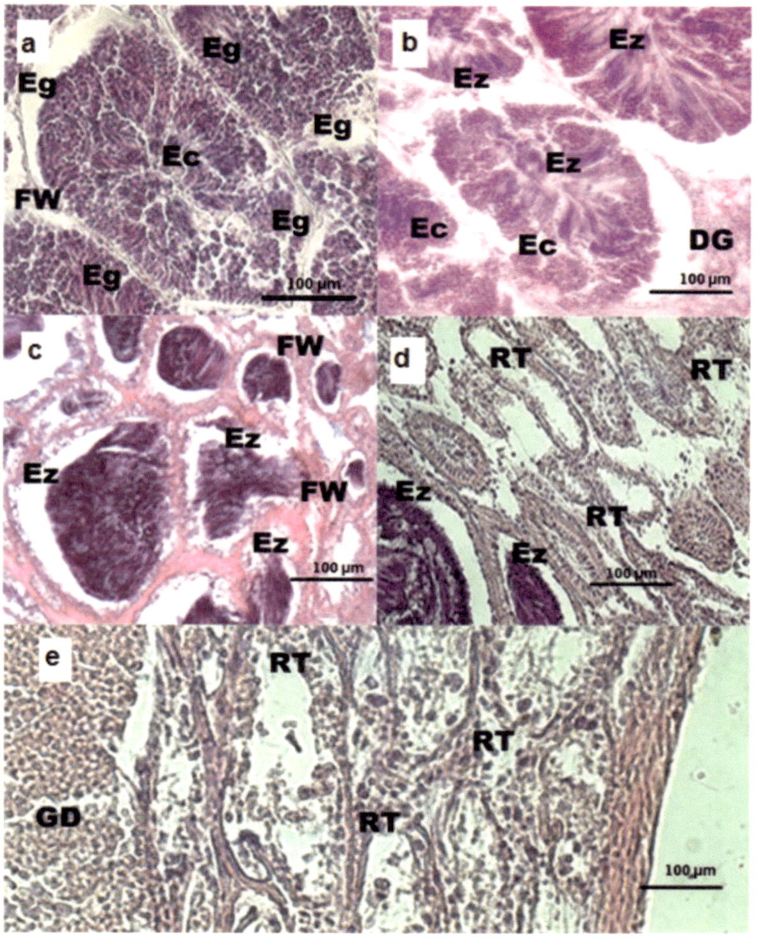

Figure 3.
Histological sections of Hexaplex princeps males showing testis stages. a: initial spermatogenesis (50 µm), b: mature (100 µm), c: spawning (10x), d: onset of rest (100 µm), e: resting (50 µm). Eg: spermatogonia, Ec: spermatocytes, Ez: spermatozoa, RS: residual spermatozoa, DG: digestive gland, CT: connective tissue, P: phagocytes.

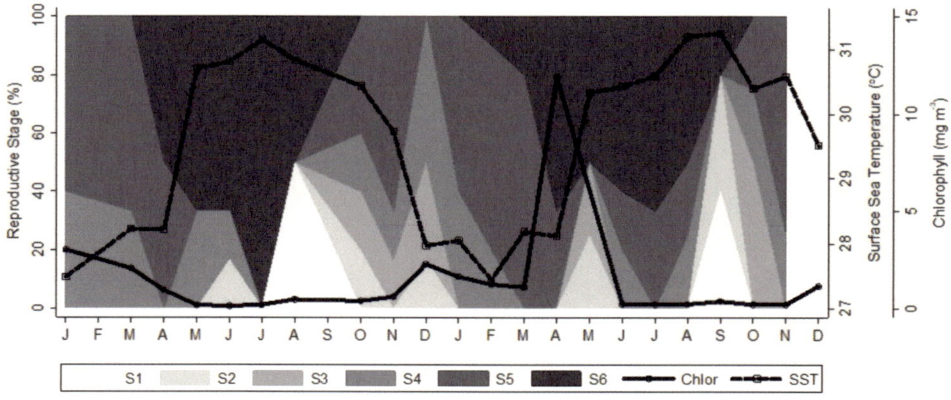

Figure 4.
Gonad stage frequency 2014–2015 for H. princeps females by sampling date. Chlorophyll concentration (mg m^{-3}) and Surface Water Temperature (°C) values are showed.

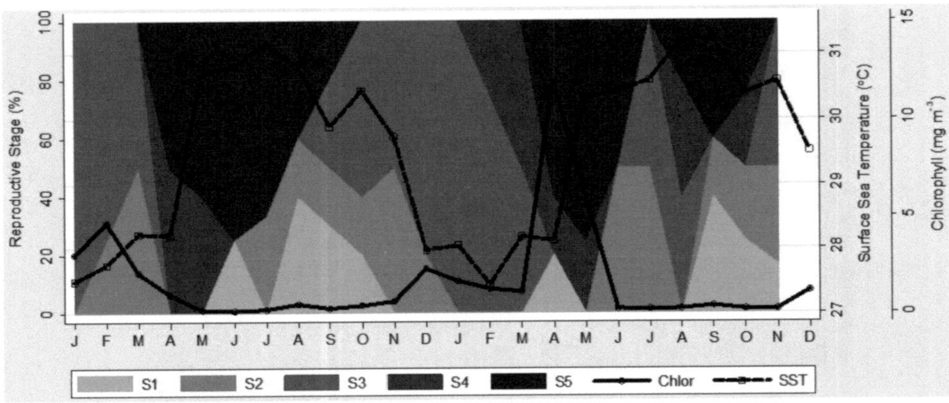

Figure 5.
Gonad stage frequency 2014–2015 for H. princeps males by sampling date. Chlorophyll concentration (mg m^{-3}) and temperature (°C) are included.

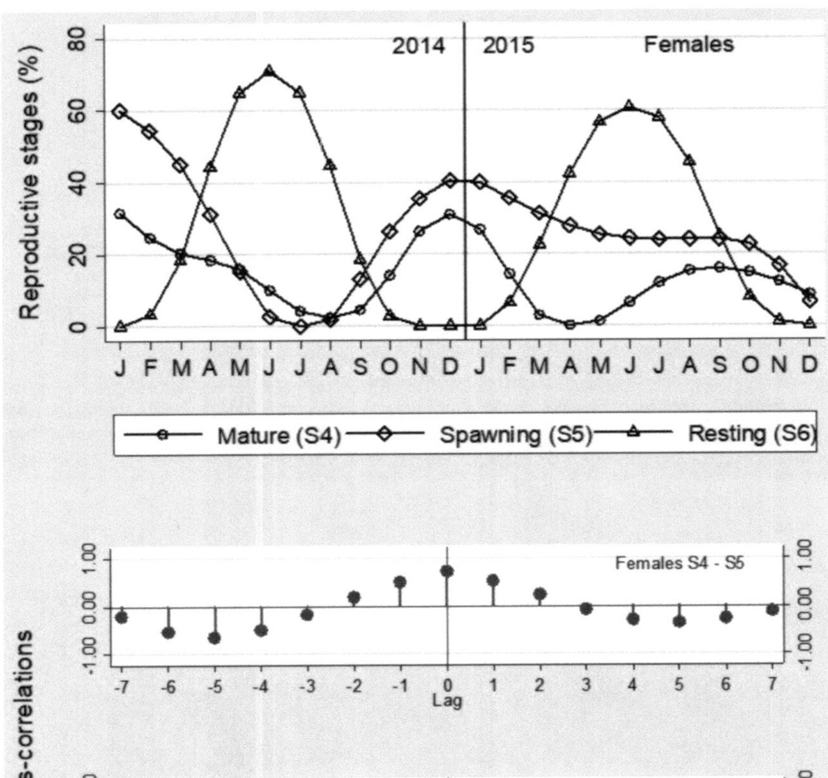

Figure 6.
The smoothed frequency of the female reproductive stages along the study period and cross-correlation correlograms for mature-spawning (S4-S5) and spawning-resting (S5-S6) reproductive stages comparison.

May (60%), June (75%), and July (67%) 2014. The months of 2015 with larger spawning (S3) percentages were January (100%) and March (50%); finally, the months with the larger frequency of resting individuals (S5) were May (60%) and June (75%).

3.2 Chlorophyll *a* concentration and gonad cycle

In 2014, the highest chlorophyll *a* concentrations were observed in January (3.00 mg m^{-3}), February (4.00 mg m^{-3}), March (2.05 mg m^{-3}), and December (2.27 mg m^{-3}); in the same months, the larger frequency of individuals in the spawning stages (S5 females, S3 males) (**Figures 4** and **5**) was observed. For the same year, low chlorophyll concentrations were recorded in June (0.15 mg m^{-3}) and July (1.10 mg m^{-3}) months, which correspond with the larger frequency of females and males in the resting stages (S6 and S5, respectively) (**Figures 4** and 5).

In 2015, the high chlorophyll concentrations were observed in January (1.62 mg m^{-3}), February (1.23 mg m^{-3}), March (1.08 mg m^{-3}), and (exceptionally) April (11.89 mg m^{-3}); except for April, in all other months, the stage with

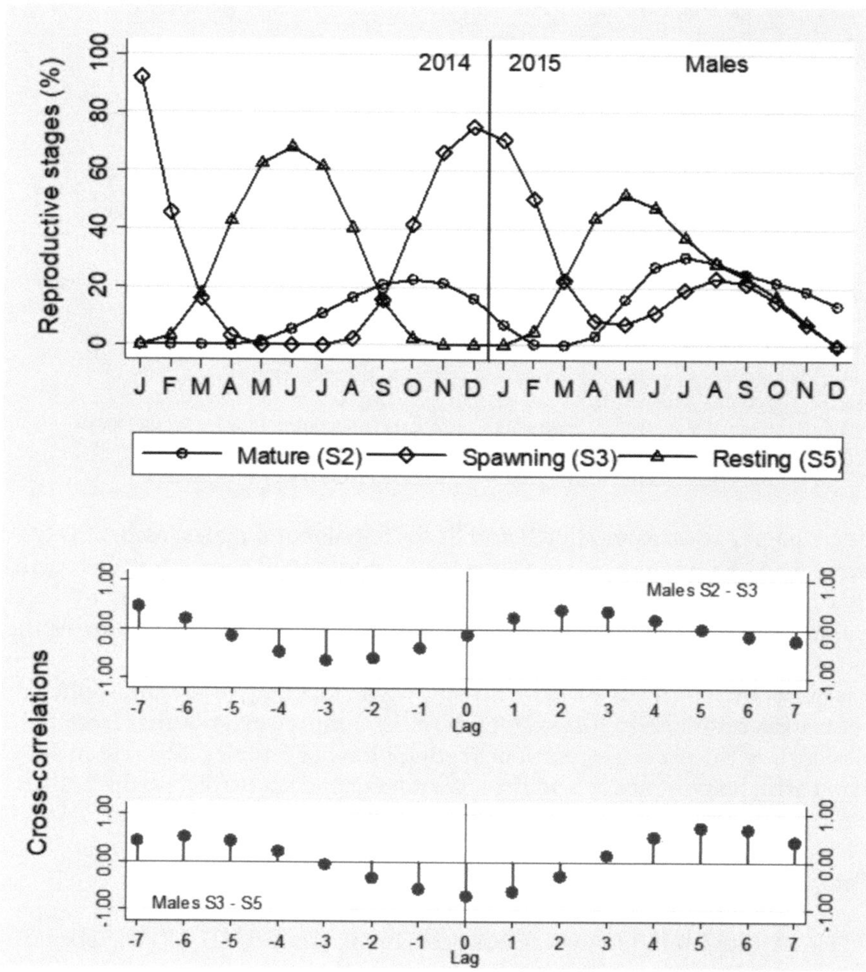

Figure 7.
The smoothed frequency of the male reproductive stages along the study period and cross-correlation correlograms for mature-spawning (S2-S3) and spawning-resting (S3-S5) reproductive stages comparison.

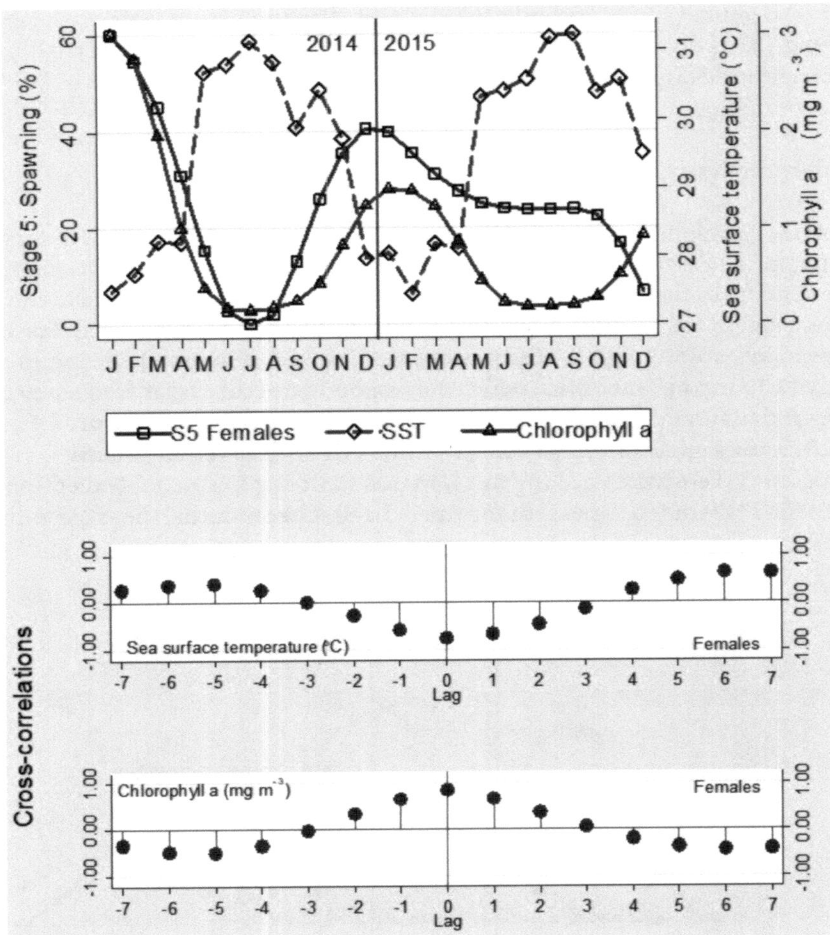

Figure 8.
The smoothed frequency of spawning females (S5), surface sea temperature (SST) and chlorophyll concentration (CL) along the study period and cross-correlation correlograms for S5-SST and S5-CL comparison.

larger frequency was spawning (S5 and S3 for females and males, respectively) (**Figures 4** and 5). In the same year, the lower chlorophyll concentrations occurred in July (0.18 mg m^{-3}), October (0.18 mg m^{-3}), and November (0.19 mg m^{-3}). These chlorophyll concentration values were related to the resting stage of females and males (S6 and S5, respectively) (**Figures 4** and 5).

It is possible that the April 2015, notably high (11.89 mg m^{-3}), chlorophyll concentration originated a different pattern, in comparison with that from the same month of the previous year. The resting phase of females (S6) and males (S5) occurred with less frequency and the spawning gonad stage (S5 females and S3 males) extended to June, July, and August (**Figures 4** and 5).

3.3 Temperature and gonad cycle

The lowest registered temperatures occurred in January (27.48°C), February (27.74°C), and December (27.96°C). In these months, it was observed that the spawning females (S6) and males (S3) were those with the highest frequency (**Figures 4** and 5). The months with the highest temperatures were May (30.70°C),

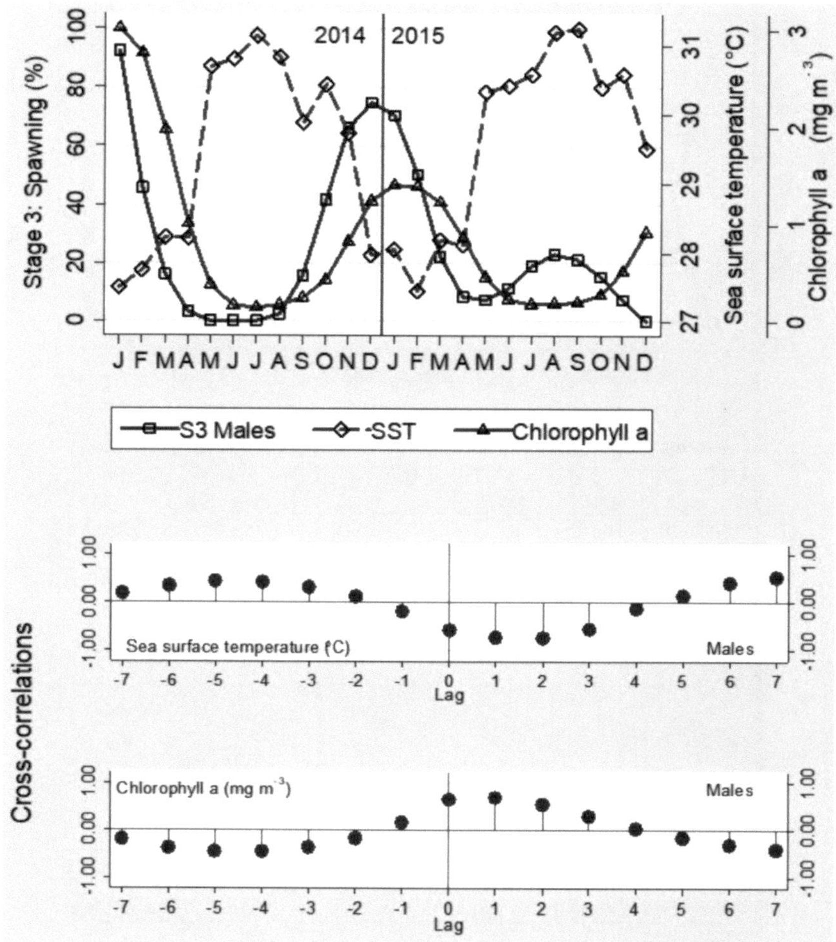

Figure 9.
The smoothed frequency of spawning males (S3), surface sea temperature (SST) and chlorophyll concentration (CL) along the study period and cross-correlation correlograms for S3-SST and S3-CL comparison.

June (31.14°C), and August (30.83°C), which were related to the larger frequency of the resting stages of females (S6) and males (S5) (**Figures 4** and **5**).

The lowest temperatures for 2015 were registered in January (28.04°C), February (27.44°C), and March (28.11°C), which corresponded with the highest frequencies of female and male in the spawning stage (S5 and S3, respectively). The months with the larger temperature values were August (31.19°C) and September (31.24°C). In these months, female stage 4 (mature), 5 (spawning), and 6 (resting) were observed with 25, 25, and 50%, respectively; the male stages were 3 (spawning) and 4 (end of spawning, onset of the rest) (50 and 30%, respectively), and in September, 35% of stage 2 (maturity), 25% of phase 3 (spawning), and 40% of stage 5 (resting) were observed.

3.4 Smoothing and cross-correlation

To describe in more detail the variation and relationships of the reproduction stages and the environmental variables, sea surface temperature (SST) and chlorophyll *a* (Cl) concentrations, along the study period, the smoothed frequency of the reproductive stages were analyzed by cross-correlation. It can be easily seen

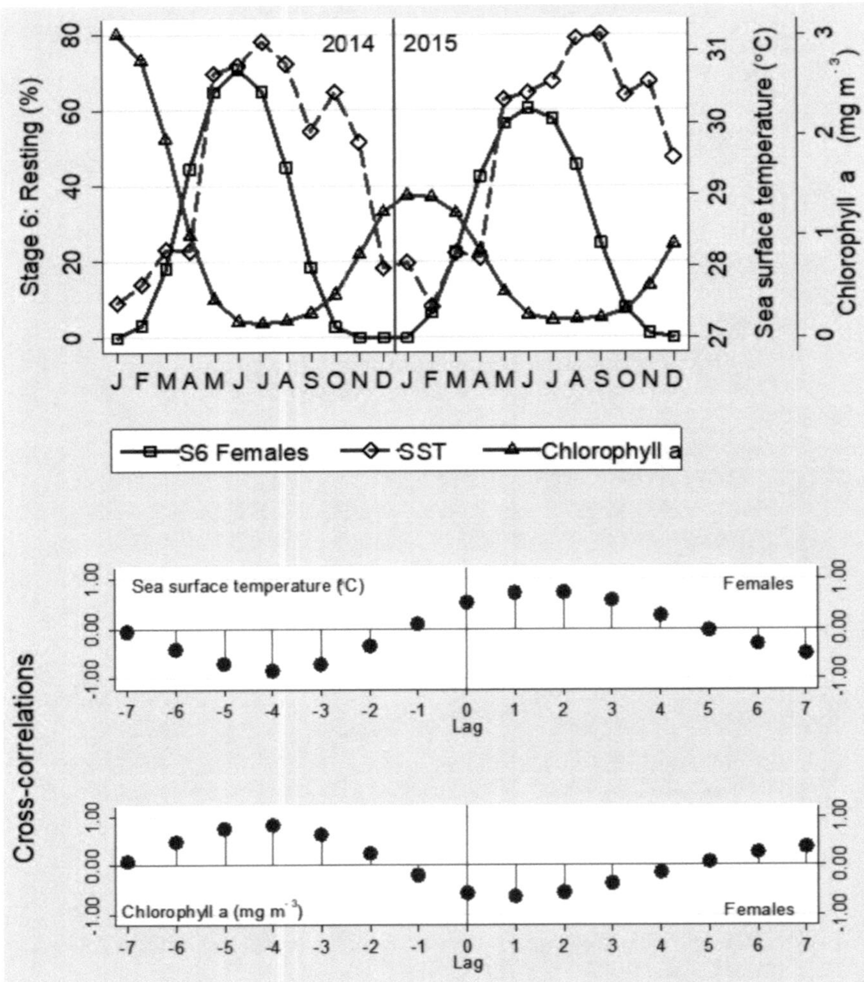

Figure 10.
The smoothed frequency of resting females (S6), surface sea temperature (SST) and chlorophyll concentration (CL) along the study period and cross-correlation correlograms for S6-SST and S6-CL comparison.

(**Figure 6**) that during the cool months of the year (from October to February), the females mature (S4) and spawn (S5) from October to March. During 2015, the spawning period lasted longer than the previous year. Very clearly, the females are in reproductive rest (S6) during the warmer half of the year (from April to August). The cross-correlation of the series shows a significant positive trend between S4 and S5 stages synchronically and an inverse correlation with 4–5 months lag between spawning (S5) and rest (S6).

The males seem to mature (S2) early (July) but the trend is clear from September to January (**Figure 7**). The spawning males (S3) occur from October to February. Similarly than females, males attain the reproductive rest stage (S5) from April to August, during the warmer months.

The cross-correlograms show a direct relationship lagged 2 months between S2 and S3 (maturity, spawning stage) and a 6 month lagged high cross-correlation between spawning (S3) and resting (S5) males, corroborating significantly the above statements.

The spawning (S5) females showed a clear opposite (negative) correlation with the sea surface temperature values with a lag of 6 months, and concordant

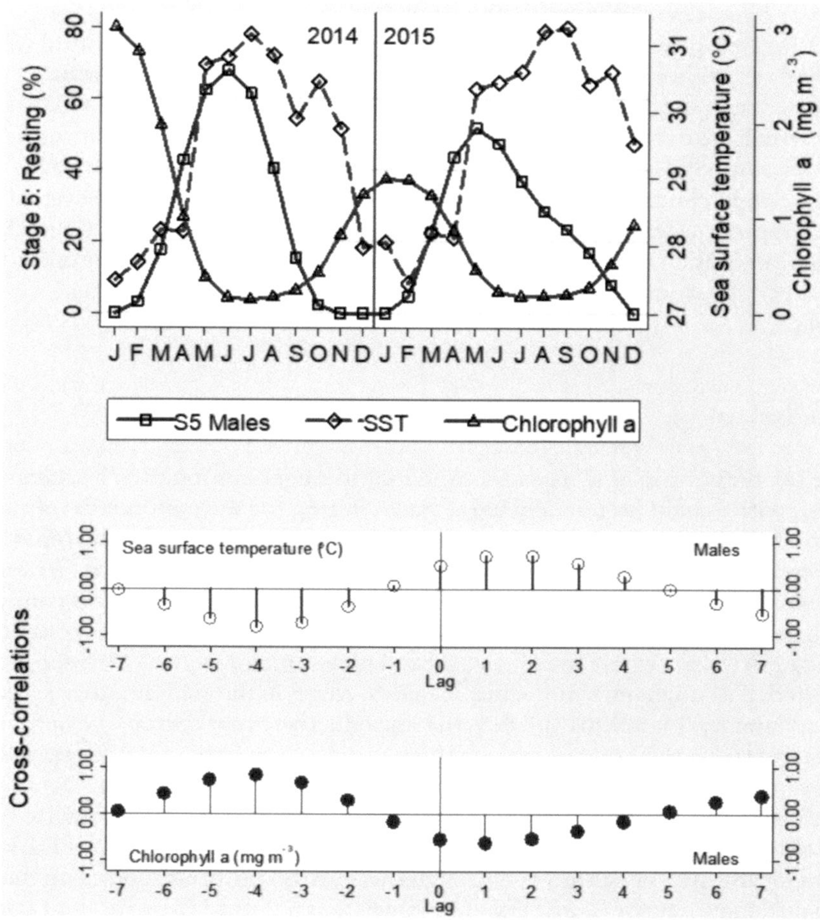

Figure 11.
The smoothed frequency of resting males (S5), surface sea temperature (SST) and chlorophyll concentration (CL) along the study period and cross-correlation correlograms for S5-SST and S5-CL comparison.

Sex	Sequence	Lag	Cross-correlation	*P*-value
Females	S4-S5	0	0.7144	0.0001
	S5-S6	4	0.7525	0.0000
Males	S2-S3	2	0.4165	0.0182
	S3-S5	5	0.7192	0.0000
Females	S5-SST	6	0.6278	0.0001
	S5-CL	0	0.8442	0.0000
Males	S3-SST	7	0.5366	0.0013
	S3-CL	1	0.6835	0.0000
Females	S6-SST	2	0.7281	0.0000
	S6-CL	−4	0.8384	0.0000
Males	S5-SST	2	0.7159	0.0000
	S5-CL	−4	0.8467	0.0000

Table 5.
Cross-correlation analysis results resume: sex, sequences compared, time lag (month), cross-correlation, and significance values.

(positive) cross-correlation with chlorophyll *a* concentration with no lag (**Figure 8**). In **Figure 9**, it is possible to see that, as the females, spawning (S3) males had negative cross-correlation values with SST values (lagged around 7 months), and positive with chlorophyll (1-month lag). In contrast with the former trends, the resting females (S6) showed positive cross-correlations (lagged 2 months) with SST and negative relationship (with a lag of 7 months) with the chlorophyll concentrations (**Figure 10**). In a similar way as resting females, males in reproductive rest stage (S5) showed a direct trend with SST (lagged 1 or 2 months) and the opposite of the chlorophyll values (a lag of 7 months) (**Figure 11**). A resume of the cross-correlations significances is included in **Table 5**.

4. Discussion

The sex proportion of *H. princeps* from Puerto Ángel was found to be statistically balanced with a slight preponderance of males during the warmer months of the year. These findings correspond with the study of Vasconcelos *et al.* [36], who reported a balanced sex ratio and males dominating among smaller individuals of *Hexaplex* (*Truncularíopsis*) *trunculus* in the Ria Formosa Lagoon in Portugal. This is contrary to the unbalanced sex ratio reported by Elhasni *et al.* [4] for *Bolinus brandaris* (another Muricid) in Tunisia, where females surpassed males, mainly during the reproduction period. Although not significant, at Puerto Ángel in the cold months (January 2014 and January, March 2015), when the reproductive event occurs, the number of females was larger than that of males, which may be associated with the reproductive behavior of this species as the females tend to aggregate for oviposition.

The histological examination of the gonads of *Hexaplex princeps* at Puerto Ángel permitted to characterize six stages of maturity development in females (**Table 3**) and five for the males (**Table 4**). Although there are no previous reports on the histological maturity for *H. princeps*, the stages characterized in the present study for the females correspond closely to those suggested for *H. trunculus* from Portugal [36]. In the case of male maturity and based on our observations of the histological sections, we consider that only five stages are enough to describe the spermatogenic cycle.

Comparing both sexes, spawning and expulsion occurred in January, April, May, October, and November, and the larger frequency of resting individuals was registered in June and July. In this way, it is possible to recognize a period of spawning and expulsion from November to March with pikes in January and February. The resting period of females occurred from March to October, with peaks in July (2014) and April–July (2015), and the males presented high resting frequency values in June (2014) and May (2015). This does not corresponds to the reproduction times reported for *H. erythrostomus* from Bahía Concepción, Baja California Sur, where the reproductive events were annotated during the warmer months (May–July) [37]; though it has to be noted that the highest temperature of 28°C of the Bahía Concepción sea surface water temperature corresponds with the cooler temperatures of Puerto Ángel. The temperature is one of the most important external environmental factors that affects molluscan reproduction and in the case of *H. princeps*, for both sexes, the spawning and expulsion stages occurred at relatively low temperatures and the resting period at warmer temperatures of surface waters at the studied locality.

Chlorophyll concentrations have a direct relationship with the development of gonads as this reproductive process demands high energetic quantities that must be obtained from the eaten food extracted from the environment or from reserves previously accumulated or from both [6, 38]. *H. princeps* is a predator gastropod that depends on the energy obtained from its preys. So, during 2014, for the females, it was noted that when the chlorophyll *a* concentrations were high, maturity and spawning stages presented a higher occurrence percentage and when the concentrations were low, the most frequent gonad stage is resting. For the males, when the chlorophyll concentrations were high, the most frequent gonad stage was the expulsion and when low concentrations occurred, the most frequent gonad stage was resting. In 2015, chlorophyll concentrations were very variable having high values from January to March and an increment in November corresponding with larger percentages of spawning females and expulsing males. However, an anomalous high peak of chlorophyll concentration occurred in April when, unlike the same month from 2014, could have caused the reduction of the resting stage and oogenesis and spermatogenesis occurred as indicated by presence of the spawning stage. Therefore, the periods with large chlorophyll availability coincide with the gonad development. *H. princeps* tends to reproduce when the phytoplankton population is blooming, so its offspring could have a higher probability of survival due to food abundance [14, 15].

In relation to temperature is worth to mention that along the period of study, the water temperature differences between surface-bottom lectures were not detected. The direct explanation for this finding is that the rocky coast localities where the individuals of *H. princeps* were collected are places very energetic under the effects of strong wave action, precisely the zones usually inhabited by this organism [7, 8].

In this study, the predominance of reproductive stages occurred during the winter months under relatively colder temperatures. As noted before, the reproduction of the related species *H. erythrostomus* in the Gulf of California happened when the water temperature was around 28°C [37], figure similar to the January surface temperatures of Puerto Ángel.

From October to April but mainly from November to February, the blowing winds, known as the "Tehuanos," originate upwelling and water vertical mixing causing an increase in chlorophyll concentrations [39, 40] by phytoplanktonic blooming. This water mixing process promotes spawning, breeding, and feeding of the aquatic species [41]. Thus, it is possible that the food availability is the main factor affecting the onset of reproduction of *H. princeps* in this region.

On the other side, we would like to mention that the smoothing technique applied to the maturity stage frequencies allow distinguishing in a clearer way the subjacent pattern of the reproductive cycle. With the availability of long-term data records, it is possible to use time series analysis statistical techniques, making it possible to assess the significance of the observed behaviors. From this, it can be stated that *H. princeps* matures and spawns during the cold months of the year (October–March) and rest its reproduction during the warm part of the year (May–August). It observed a positive correlation with the quantity of food (indirectly indicated by the chlorophyll *a* concentrations) and in all the cases, the leads and lags of these variables can be determined [35].

This is the first study on the reproductive cycle of *H. princeps* in the region and present baseline information for: (i) potential management measures, in particular, the knowledge of the timing of spawning season, (ii) assessment of aquaculture potential. More research on the subject is needed.

5. Conclusions

The reproductive cycle of *Hexaplex princeps* was studied through monthly histological analysis of gonads during two annual periods (2014, 2015) from specimens obtained from the artisanal fishery at Puerto Ángel, Oaxaca, Mexico, considering sexual proportion, gonad maturation, spawning periods, and maturity stages variation in relation with environmental factors (sea surface temperature and chlorophyll concentration).

The sexual proportion was not statistically different from parity, although most of the times, the number of males was slightly larger than the number of females. Only during the spawning season, females were more frequent than males.

The histological analysis permitted to establish maturity stages.

Females (six stages): (1) initial oogenesis, (2) previtellogenic maturity, (3) vitellogenic maturity, (4) maturity, (5) spawning, and (6) resting.

Males (five stages): (1) initial spermatogenesis, (2) maturity, (3) spawning, (4) onset of the rest, and (5) resting.

Monthly variations of maturation stages showed that *H. princeps* has an annual reproductive cycle with a long period of gonadal activity. The spawning season comprised from November to March (females) and from December to March (males) with activity peaks in January. From March to October (females) and May to June (males) reproduction resting occurred.

Reproductive events were related to high chlorophyll *a* concentrations due to the upwelling processes resulting from the predominant winds and to the relatively cooler temperatures proper to the winter (November–March) season at Puerto Ángel, Oaxaca, Mexico.

Acknowledgements

We express our thankfulness to the Posgrado en Ciencias Biológicas, Universidad Nacional Autónoma de México (UNAM), and the Consejo Nacional de Ciencia y Tecnología (CONACyT) for their support. Without the help of the local divers Manolo Jarquín, Primitivo Herrera Ordóñez and Captain "Beto" (Abraham Reyes López), the collection of specimens would not have been possible. We are grateful to Dr. Erika Rosales Cruz for her help with the histological photographs and to the Central de Instrumentación de Microscopía, Escuela Nacional de Ciencias Biológicas, Instituto Politécnico Nacional. This research received support from Dirección del Personal Académico, UNAM under the programs PAPIME (PE206213, PE207417) and (partially) PAPIIT (IG201215). Besides, we received support from the Carrera de Biología, Facultad de Estudios Superiores (FES) Zaragoza, UNAM. Lastly, we would thank all the students and colleagues of the Laboratorio de Biometría y Biología Pesquera, FES Zaragoza, UNAM. This research report is part of first author's PhD thesis.

Conflict of interest

We state that there is no "conflict of interest."

DOI: http://dx.doi.org/10.5772/intechopen.88074

Author details

Verónica Mitsui Saito-Quezada[1], Esther Uría-Galicia[2], José Luis Gómez-Márquez[3], Ana Bertha Villaseñor-Martínez[4], Ma. De Lourdes Jiménez-Badillo[5] and Isaías Hazarmabeth Salgado-Ugarte[1*]

1 Laboratorio de Biometría y Biología Pesquera, FES Zaragoza, UNAM, Mexico

2 Laboratorio de Histología, Departamento de Morfología, ENCB, IPN, Mexico

3 Laboratorio de Limnología, FES Zaragoza, UNAM, Mexico

4 Departamento de Paleontología, Instituto de Geología, UNAM, Mexico

5 Instituto de Ciencias Marinas y Pesquerías, Universidad Veracruzana, Veracruz, Mexico

*Address all correspondence to: ihsalgadougarte@gmail.com

References

[1] FAO. The Estate of World Fisheries and Aquaculture (SOFIA). Roma: United Nations Food and Agricultural Organization; 2016. Available from: http://www.fao.org/3/a-i5555e.pdf

[2] Marean CW. The origins and significance of coastal resource use in Africa and Western Eurasia. Journal of Human Evolution. 2014;**77**:17-40. DOI: 10.1016/j.jhevol.2014.02.025

[3] Leiva GE, Castilla JC. A review of the world marine gastropod fishery: Evolution of the catches, management and the Chilean experience. Reviews in Fish Biology and Fisheries. 2002;**1**:283-300. DOI: 10.1023/a:1021368216294

[4] Elhasni K, Vasconcelos P, Ghorbel M, Jarbout O. Reproductive cycle of *Bolinus brandaris* (Gastropoda: Muricidae) in the Gulf of Gabès (southern Tunisia). Aquatic Biology. 2013;**16**:69-83. DOI: 10.12681/mms.325

[5] Secretaría de Agricultura, Ganadería, Desarrollo Rural, Pesca y Alimentación (SAGARPA). Anuario Estadístico de Acuacultura y Pesca 2013 de la Comisión Nacional de Acuacultura y Pesca; Mexico2015. p. 299

[6] Fretter V. Prosobranchs. In: Tompa AS, Verdonk HH, Van Der Biggelaar J, editors. The Mollusca: Reproduction. Vol. 7. London: Academic Press; 1984. pp. 1-45

[7] Keen AM. Sea Shells of Tropical West America (Marine Mollusks from Baja California to Peru). Stanford: Stanford University Press; 1971. p. 632

[8] Morris AP. A Field Guide to Pacific Coast Shells Including Shells of Hawaii and the Gulf of California. Boston: Houghton Mifflin Company; 1976. p. 176

[9] Vega AJ, González A. Moluscos del Pacífico Veragüense, parte II (Gastropoda). Tecnociencia. 2002;**4**(1):23-45

[10] Landa-Jaime V, Michel-Morfín E, Arciniega-Flores J, Castillo-Vargasmachuca S, Saucedo-Lozano M. Moluscos asociados al arrecife coralino de Tenacatita, Jalisco, en el Pacífico central mexicano. Revista Mexicana de Biodiversidad. 2013;**84**:1121-1136. DOI: 10.7550/rmb.32994

[11] Castro-Mondragón H, Flores-Garza R, Rosas-Acevedo JL, Flores-Rodríguez P, García-Ibáñez S, Valdéz-González A. Escenario biológico pesquero y socio-económico de la pesca ribereña de moluscos en Acapulco. Revista Iberoamericana de Ciencia Tecnología y Sociedad. 2015;**2**(7):7-23. DOI: 10.15174/au.2016.1025

[12] Defeo O, Castilla JC. More than one bag for the world fishery crisis and keys for co-management successes in selected artisanal Latin American shellfisheries. Reviews in Fish Biology and Fisheries. 2005;**15**:265-283. DOI: 10.1007/s11160-005-4865-0

[13] Underwood AJ, Keough MJ. Supply-side ecology: The nature and consequences of variations in recruitment of intertidal organisms. In: Hay M, Gaines S, Bertness M, editors. Marine Community Ecology. Sunderland: Sinauer Association; 2001. pp. 183-200

[14] Varpe O, Jorgensen C, Tarling GA, Fiksen O. Early is better: Seasonal egg fitness and timing of reproduction in a zooplankton life-history model. Oikos. 2007;**116**:1331-1342. DOI: 10.1111/j.2007.0030-1299.15893.x

[15] Avaca MS, Martín P, van der Molen S, Narvarte M. Comparative study of the female gametogenic cycle in three populations of *Buccinanops globulosus* (Caenogastropoda:

Nassariidae) from Patagonia. Helgoland Marine Research. 2015;**69**:87-99. DOI: 10.1007/s10152-014-0418-z

[16] Vasconcelos P, Moura P, Barroso CM, Gaspar MB. Reproductive cycle of *Bolinus brandaris* (Gastropoda: Muricidae) in the Ria Formosa lagoon (southern Portugal). Aquatic Biology. 2012;**16**:69-83. DOI: 10.3354/ab00434

[17] Cudney-Bueno R, Prescott R, Hinojosa-Huerta O. The black murex snail, *Hexaplex nigritus* (Mollusca, Muricidae), in the Gulf of California, Mexico. I. Reproductive ecology and breeding aggregations. Bulletin of Marine Science. 2008;**83**(2):299-313

[18] Wolfson FH. Spawning notes. I. *Hexaplex erythrostomus*. The Veliger. 1968;**10**(3):292

[19] Ortíz-Ordoñez E, Mendoza-Santana EL, Belmar-Pérez J, Padilla-Benavides T. Histological description of the male and female gonads in *Tegula eiseni*, *T. funebraris*, *T. aureotincta*, *T. gallina* and *T. regina*, from Bahía Tortugas BCS, Mexico. International Journal of Morphology. 2009;**27**(3):691-697. DOI: 10.4067/s0717-95022009000300011

[20] Sokal RR, Rohlf FJ. Biometry: The Principles and Practice of Statistics in Biological Research. New York: W.H. Freeman & Co; 1995. p. 887

[21] Crawley MJ. Statistical Computing: An Introduction to Data Analysis Using S-Plus. Chichester: John Wiley & Sons; 2002. p. 184

[22] Uría-Galicia E, Mora-Vázquez C. Apuntes Para el Curso Teórico Práctico de Histología Animal. Mexico: Instituto Politécnico Nacional; 1996. p. 277

[23] Goddard Earth Sciences Data and Information Services Center, National Aeronautics and Space Administration (GES DISC—NASA). Monthly Average of the Sea Surface Temperature at Daylight, Expressed in Celsius Degrees. 2016. Raster Digital Data Available From: http://giovanni.gsfc.nasa.gov/giovanni/. Published at: http://www.icmyl.unam.mx/uninmar/ [Accessed: 01 June 2016]

[24] Goddard Earth Sciences Data and Information Services Center, National Aeronautics and Space Administration (GES DISC—NASA). Monthly Average of the Sea Surface Concentration of Chlorophyll-a, Expressed in Milligrams per Cubic Meter. 2016. Raster Digital Data Available From: http://giovanni.gsfc.nasa.gov/giovanni/. Published at: http://www.icmyl.unam.mx/uninmar/ [Accessed: 02 June 2016]

[25] Velleman PF. Definition and comparison of robust nonlinear data smoothing algorithms. Journal of the American Statistical Association. 1980;**75**(371):609-615. DOI: 10.1080/01621459.1980.10477521

[26] Velleman PF, Hoaglin DC. Applications, Basics, and Computing of Exploratory Data Analysis. Boston: Duxbury Press; 1981. pp. 41-63

[27] Goodall C. A survey of smoothing techniques. In: Fox J, Long JS, editors. Modern Methods of Data Analysis. Newbury Park: Sage Publications; 1990. pp. 58-125

[28] Gould WW. sg11.1: Quantile regression with bootstrapped standard errors. In: Stata Technical Bulletin 9: 19-21. Reprinted in Stata Technical Bulletin Reprints. Vol. 2. College Station: Stata Press; 1992. pp. 137-139

[29] Salgado-Ugarte IH. El Análisis Exploratorio de Datos Biológicos. Fundamentos y Aplicaciones. Marc Ediciones y ENEP Zaragoza UNAM: Mexico; 1992. p. 243

[30] Salgado-Ugarte IH. Métodos Estadísticos Exploratorios y Confirmatorios Para Análisis de

Datos. Un Enfoque Biométrico. Mexico: DGAPA—FES Zaragoza UNAM; 2017. p. 299. Available from: http://www.librosoa.unam.mx/handle/123456789/296

[31] Salgado-Ugarte IH, Curts-García J. sed7: Resistant smoothing using Stata. In: Stata Technical Bulletin 7: 8-11. Reprinted in Stata Technical Bulletin Reprints. Vol. 2. College Station: Stata Press; 1992. pp. 99-103

[32] Salgado-Ugarte IH, Curts-García J. sed7.2: Twice reroughing procedure for resistant nonlinear smoothing. In: Stata Technical Bulletin 11: 14-16. Reprinted in Stata Technical Bulletin Reprints. Vol. 2. College Station: Stata Press; 1993. pp. 108-111

[33] StataCorp. Stata: Release 13. Statistical Software. College Station: StataCorp LP; 2013. pp. 2183-2190

[34] Davis JC. Statistics and Data Analysis in Geology. Nueva York: John Wiley & Sons; 2002. p. 638

[35] Becketti S. Introduction to Time Series Using Stata. College Station: Stata Press; 2013. p. 443

[36] Vasconcelos P, Lopes B, Castro M, Gaspar MB. Gametogenic cycle of *Hexaplex* (*Trunculariopsis*) *trunculus* (Gastropoda: Muricidae) in the Ria Formosa lagoon (Algarve coast, southern Portugal). Journal of the Marine Biological Association of the United Kingdom. 2008;**82**:321-329. DOI: 10.1017/s0025315408000593

[37] Baqueiro-Cárdenas E, Massó-Rojas JA, Vélez-Barajas A. Crecimiento y reproducción de una población de caracol chino *Hexaplex erythrostomus* (Swainson, 1831) de Bahía Concepción, B.C.S. Ciencia Pesquera. 1983;**4**:19-31

[38] García-Domínguez FA, De Haro-Hernández A, García-Cuellar A, Villalejo-Fuerte M, Rodríguez-Astudillo S. Ciclo reproductivo de *Anasara tuberculosa* (Sowerby, 1833) (Arcidae) en Bahía Magdalena, México. Revista de Biología Marina y Oceanografía. 2008;**43**(1):143-152

[39] Barton DE, Argote ML, Brown J, Kosro MP, Lavin M, Robles JM, et al. Super squirt: Dynamics of the Gulf of Tehuantepec, Mexico. Oceanography. 1993;**6**:23-30

[40] Trasviña A, Barton ED. Los nortes del golfo de tehuantepec: Dinámica del océano costero. In: Lavin MF, editor. Contribuciones a la Oceanografía Física en México, Monografía No. 3; Unión Geofísica Mexicana. 1997. pp. 25-46

[41] Alejo-Plata MC. Biología del dorado *Coryphaena hippurus* (Linnaeus, 1758) y sus implicaciones para la pesquería artesanal del Pacífico Sur de México [PhD thesis]. Mexico: Universidad Nacional Autónoma de México; 2012